STUDENT WORKBOOK FOR

ILLUSTRATED

Dental Embryology, Histology, AND Anatomy

FOURTH EDITION

MARGARET J. FEHRENBACH, RDH, MS

Oral Biologist and Dental Hygienist
Adjunct Instructor, Bachelor of Applied Science Degree Dental Hygiene Program,
Seattle Central College, Seattle, Washington
Educational Consultant and Dental Science Technical Writer,
Seattle, Washington

ELSEVIER

ELSEVIER

3251 Riverport Lane
St. Louis, Missouri 63043

**STUDENT WORKBOOK FOR ILLUSTRATED DENTAL
EMBRYOLOGY, HISTOLOGY AND ANATOMY, FOURTH EDITION** ISBN: 978-1-4557-7645-0

Content Strategist: Kristin Wilhelm
Content Development Manager: Ellen Wurm-Cutter
Content Development Specialist: Katie Gutierrez
Publishing Services Manager: Hemamalini Rajendrababu
Project Manager: Kamatchi Madhavan
Design Direction: Ashley Miner
Cover Designer: Venkatram Gopalakrishnan

Printed in the United States of America

Last digit is the print number: 9 8 7 6 5 4 3 2 1

PREFACE

This companion to *Illustrated Dental Embryology, Histology, and Anatomy* provides a wide range of activities and skill-building exercises to strengthen the student dental professional's understanding of the principles discussed in the main textbook. This workbook features activities such as structure identification exercises, glossary exercises, tooth drawing exercises, infection control guidelines for extracted teeth, and review questions. Patient examination procedures for extraoral and intraoral structures, the dentition, and occlusal evaluation have been added to integrate the clinical information with the basic science information within the included clinical exercises. Case studies are also included as well as removable flashcards using the original illustrations of the permanent dentition from the textbook.

Additional material for students can be found online on the associated Evolve website, including answers to the Workbook's glossary exercises and review questions. We hope that this material will help students integrate their knowledge more easily into clinical dental coursework.

Margaret J. Fehrenbach

CONTENTS

Note: Answers can be obtained from comparing your fill-ins to the labels on numbered figures from the textbook. Feel free to add additional labeling as you want and other notations.

UNIT I: OROFACIAL STRUCTURES

Chapter 1: Face and Neck Regions

1. Figure 1-1

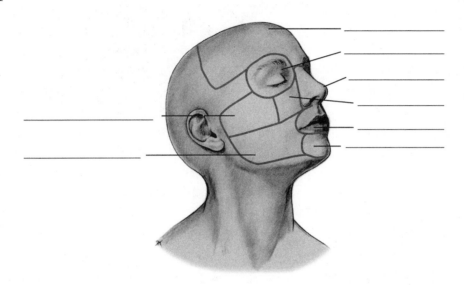

2. Figure 1-11

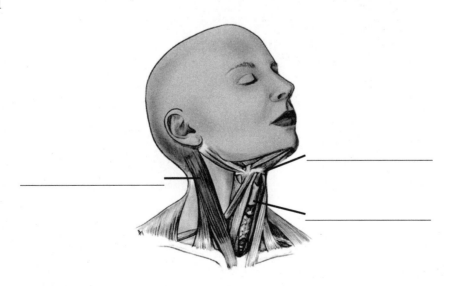

3. Figure 1-2, *A, B*

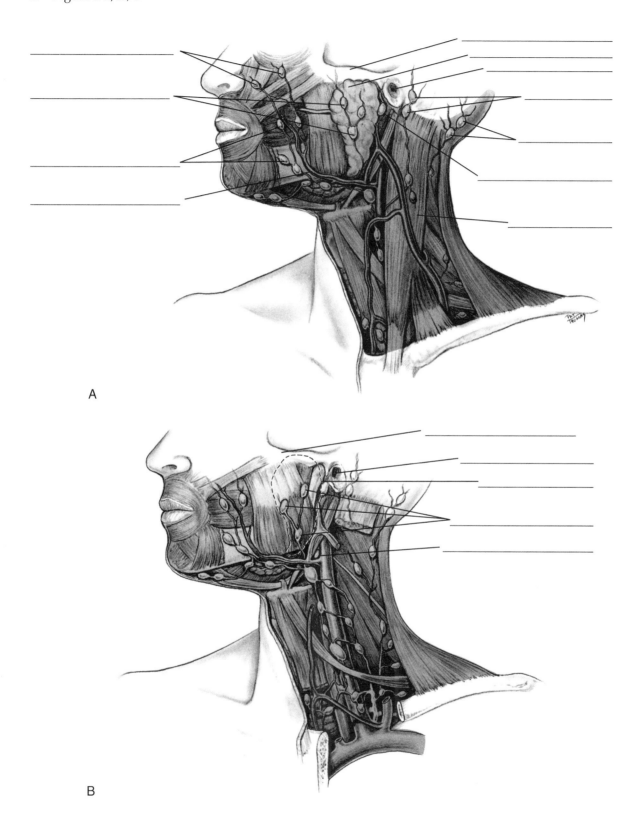

A

B

4. Figure 1-5

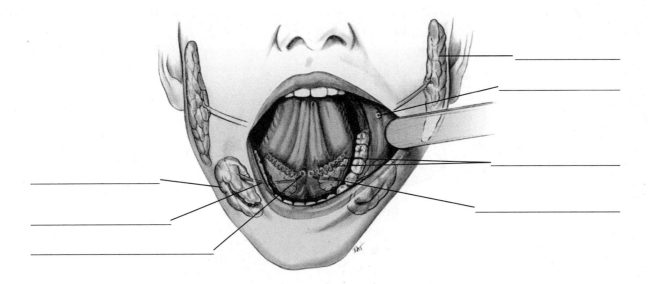

5. Figure 1-13

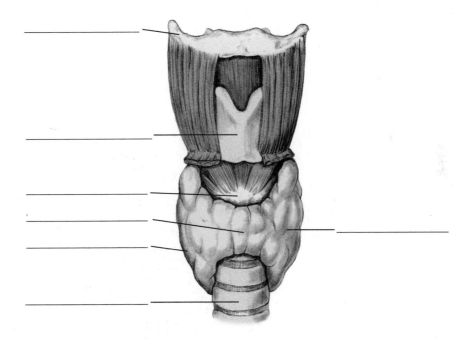

6. Figure 1-12, *A, B*

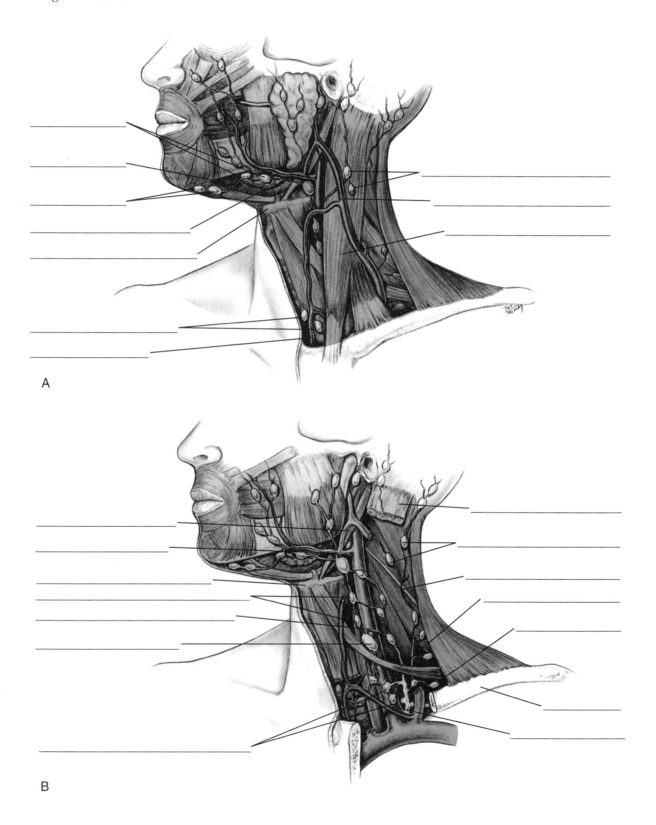

A

B

Chapter 2: Oral Cavity and Pharynx

1. Figure 2-1

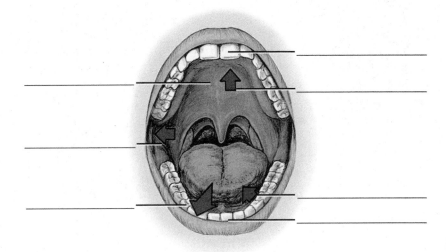

2. Figure 2-4

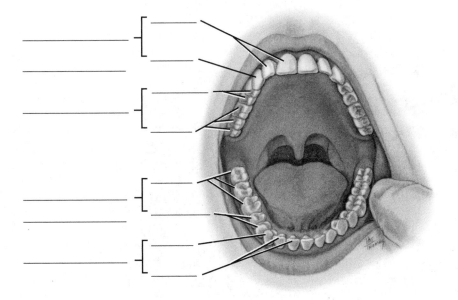

3. Figure 2-6

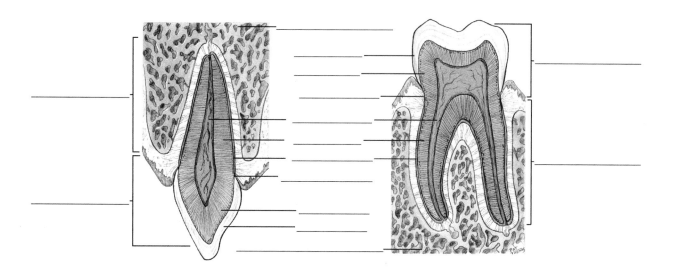

4. Figure 2-11

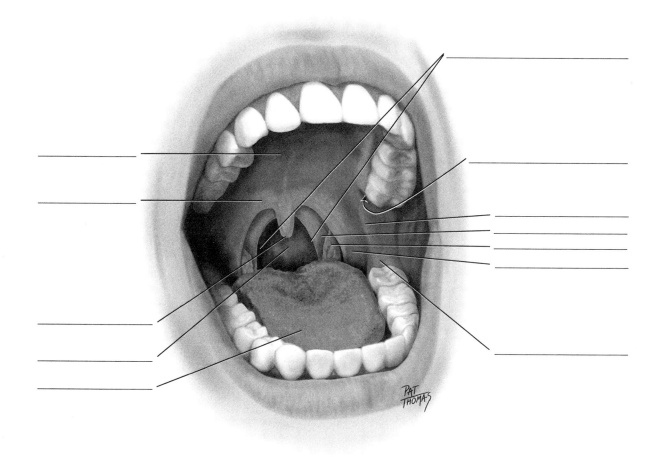

5. Figure 2-14, *A*

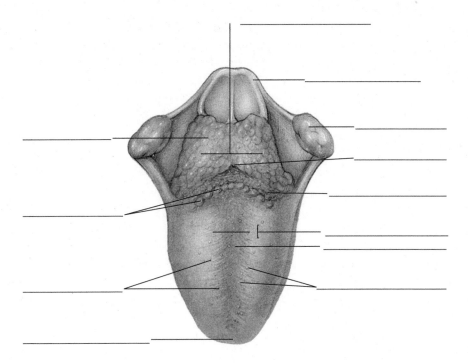

6. Figure 2-18

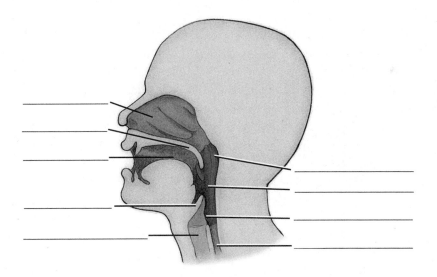

UNIT II: DENTAL EMBRYOLOGY

Chapter 3: Prenatal Development

1. Figure 3-4, *B*

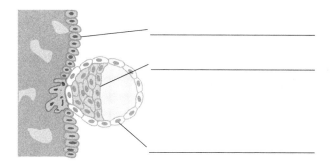

2. Figure 3-6, *A*

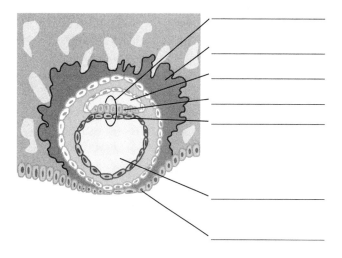

3. Figure 3-7

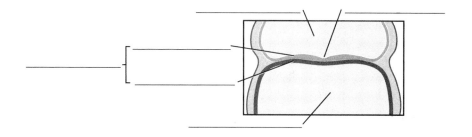

4. Figure 3-8

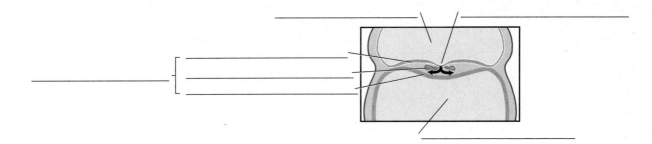

5. Figure 3-9

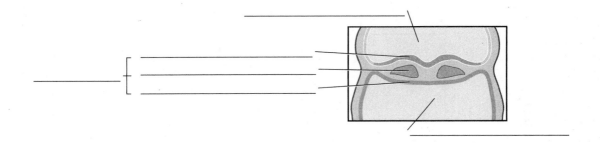

6. Figure 3-10, *A, B, C*

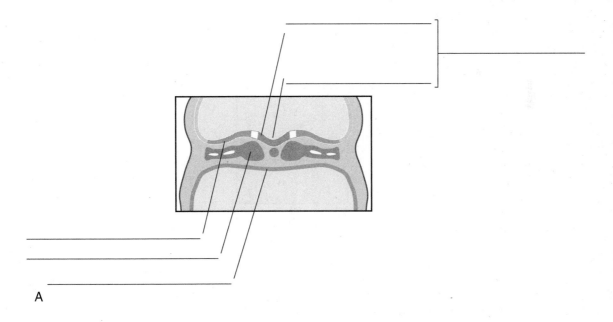

A

6. Figure 3-10, *A, B, C* (continued)

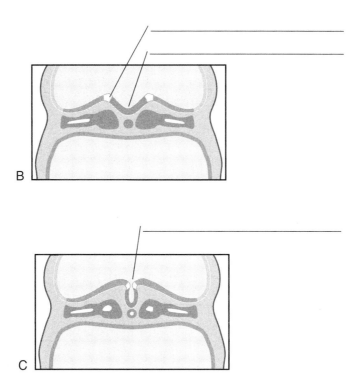

7. Figure 3-12, *A, B*

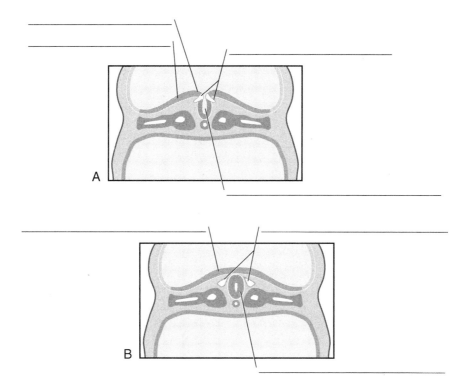

8.   Figure 3-14, *B, C*

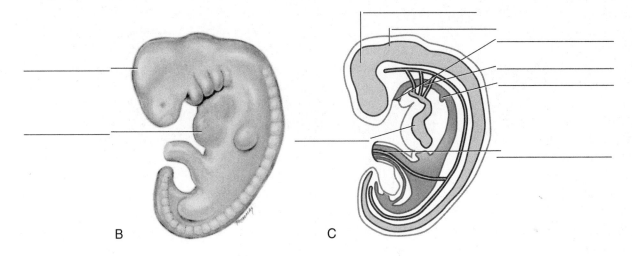

B   C

Chapter 4: Face and Neck Development

9.   Figure 4-2

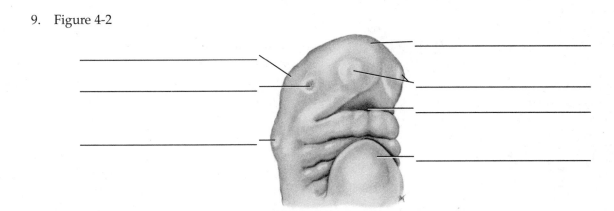

10.   Figure 4-3

Embryonic derivatives

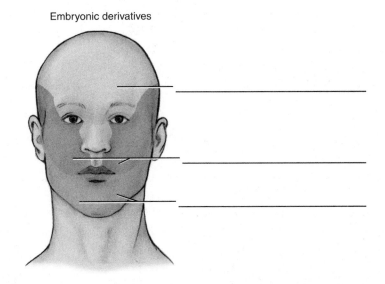

11. Figure 4-5

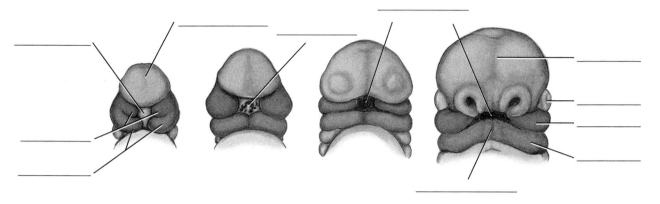

12. Figure 4-6

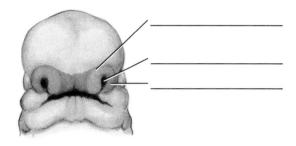

13. Figure 4-7, *B*, *C*

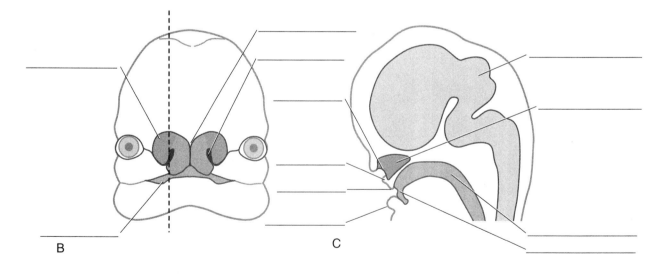

B   C

14. Figure 4-11, *B, C*

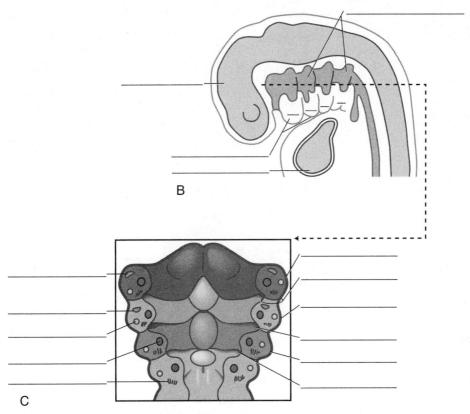

Chapter 5: Orofacial Development

15. Figure 5-1, *A, B*

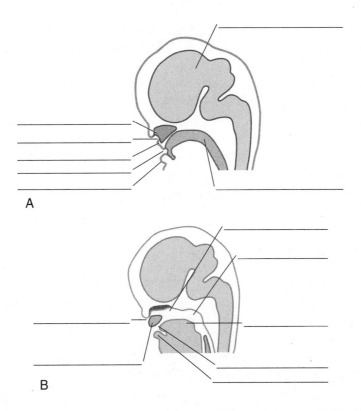

16. Figure 5-2, *A, C*

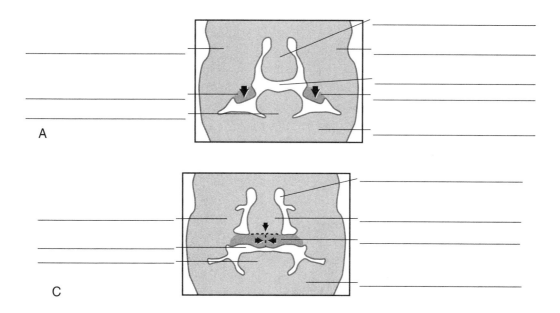

17. Figure 5-4, *B, C, D*

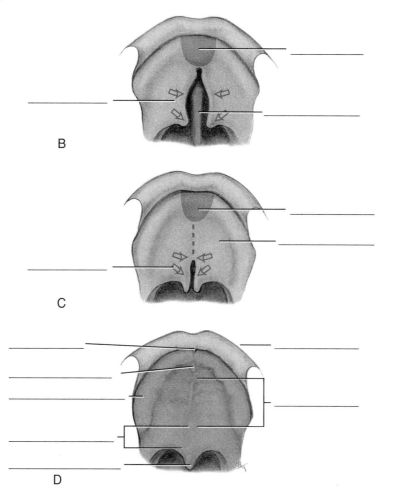

18. Figure 5-9, *A, B, C*

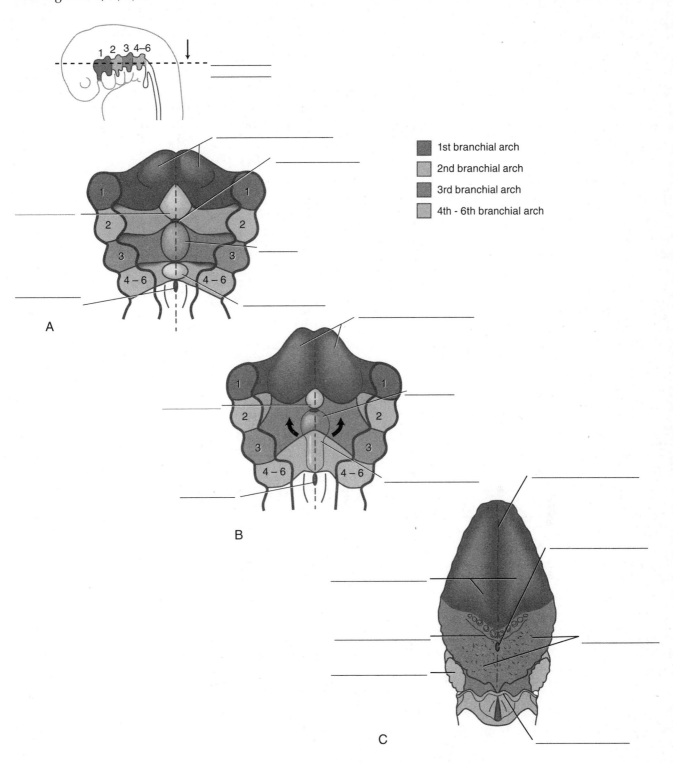

1st branchial arch

2nd branchial arch

3rd branchial arch

4th - 6th branchial arch

A

B

C

Chapter 6: Tooth Development and Eruption

19. Figure 6-2

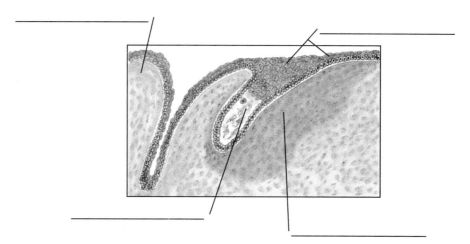

20. Figure 6-3

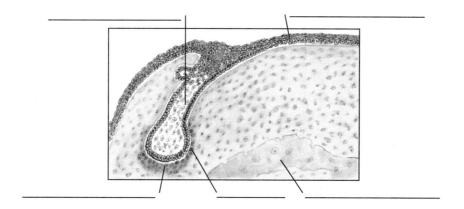

21. Figure 6-5

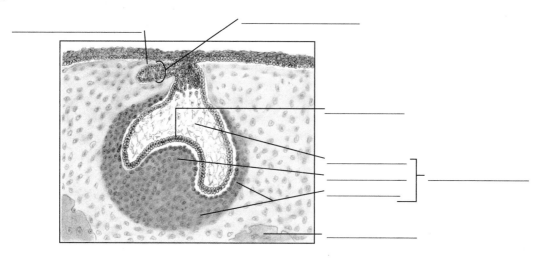

22. Figure 6-7

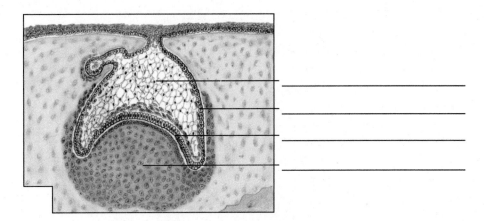

23. Figure 6-7

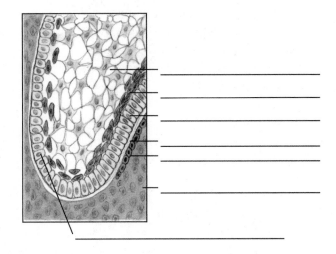

24. Figure 6-12

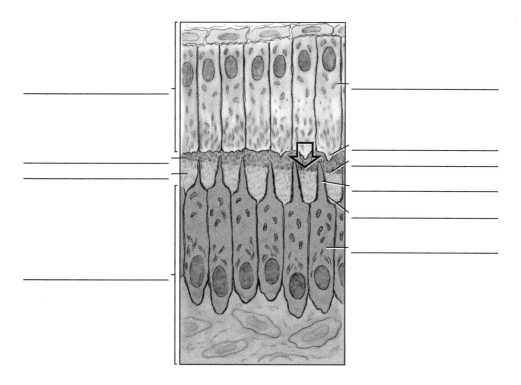

25. Figure 6-13

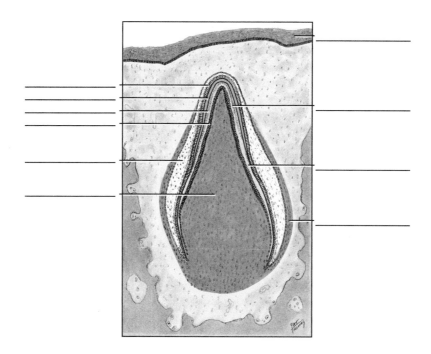

26.   Figure 6-18, *A, B*

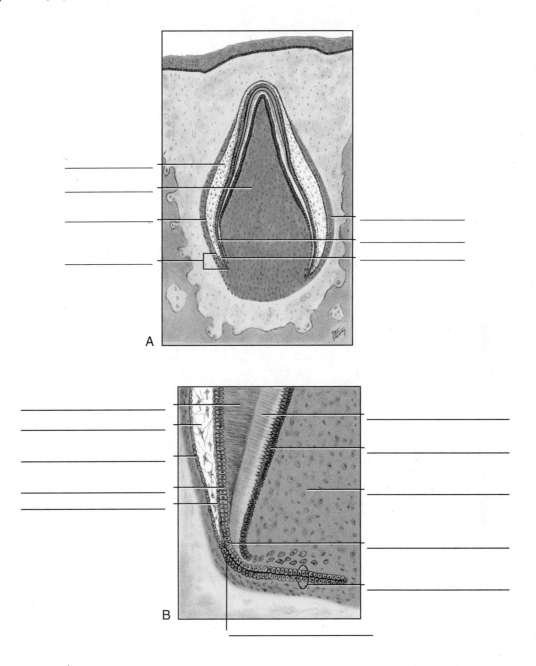

27. Figure 6-19

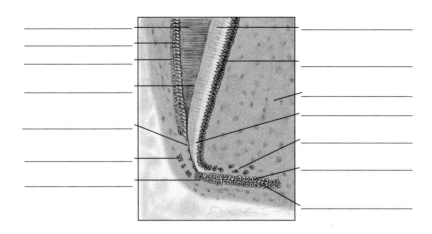

28. Figure 6-20

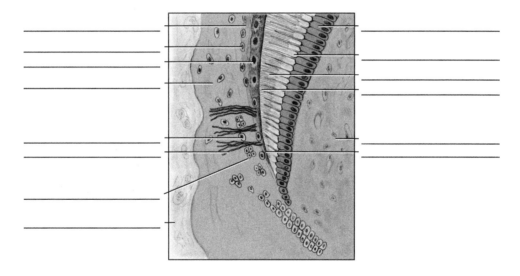

29. Figure 6-23

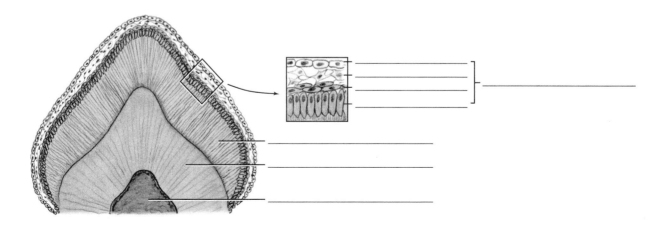

30. Figure 6-26

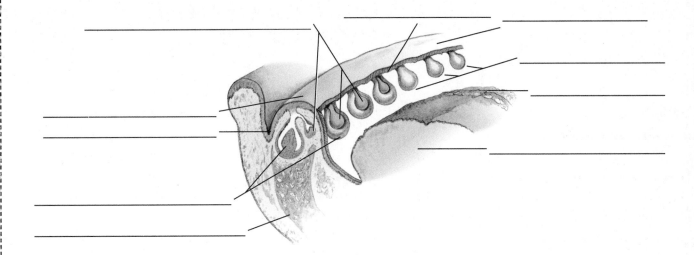

31. Figure 6-27, *B, C* (Courtesy of Margaret J. Fehrenbach, RDH, MS.)

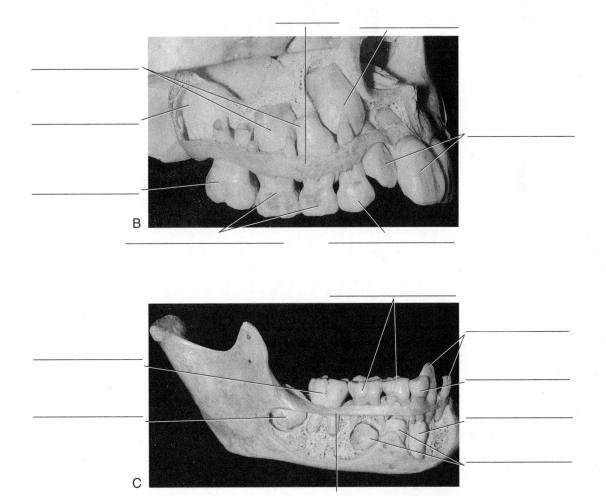

UNIT III: DENTAL HISTOLOGY

Chapter 7: Cells

1. Figure 7-2

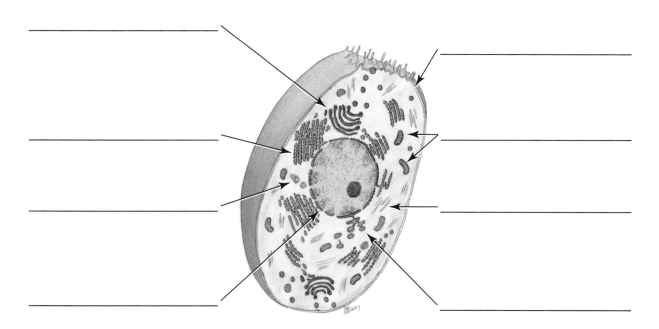

2. Figure 7-3

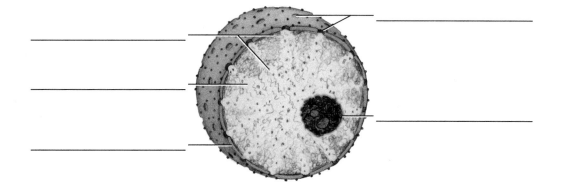

Chapter 8: Basic Tissue

3. Figure 8-4

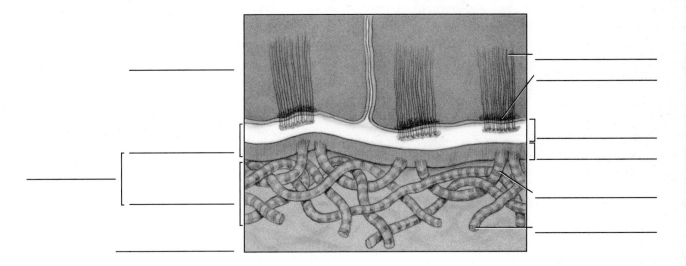

4. Figure 8-5, *A*

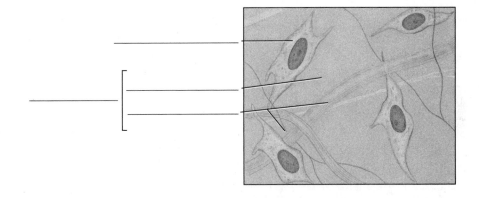

5. Figure 8-6

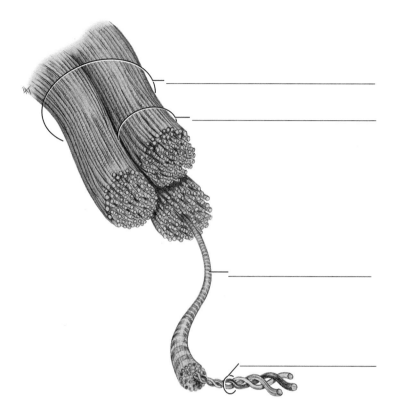

6. Figure 8-7

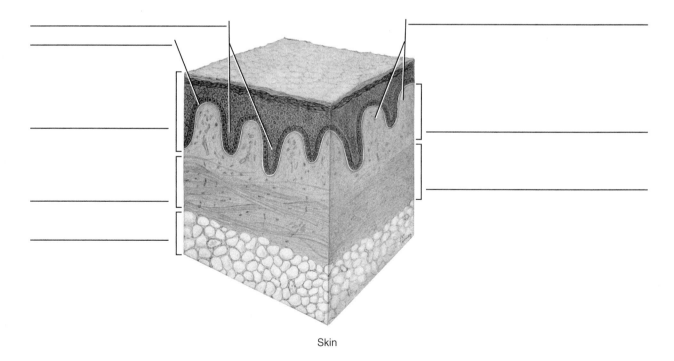

Skin

7. Figure 8-8

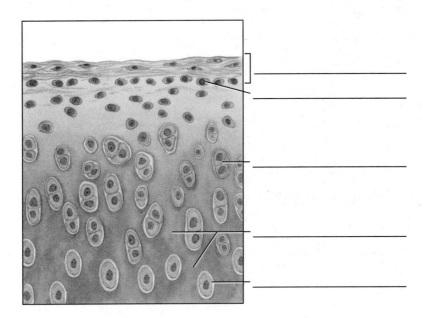

8. Figure 8-9

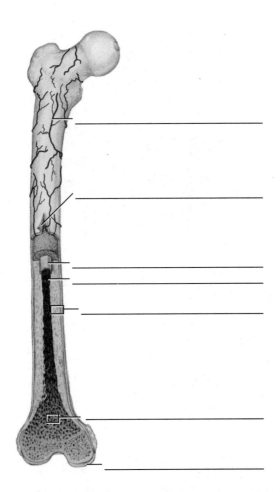

9.   Figure 8-10

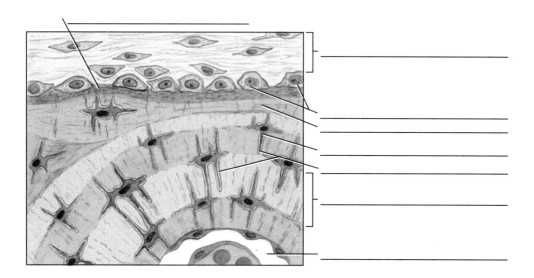

10.   Figure 8-11, *A*

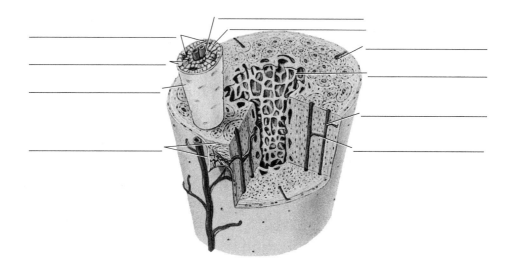

11.   Figure 8-15

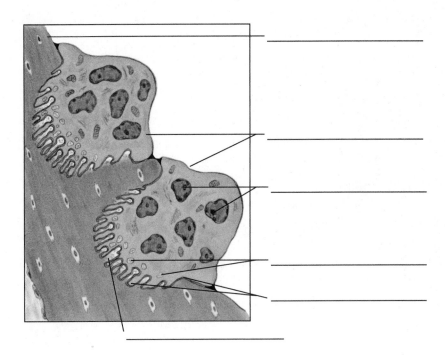

_____

_____

_____

_____

_____

_____

12.   Figure 8-18

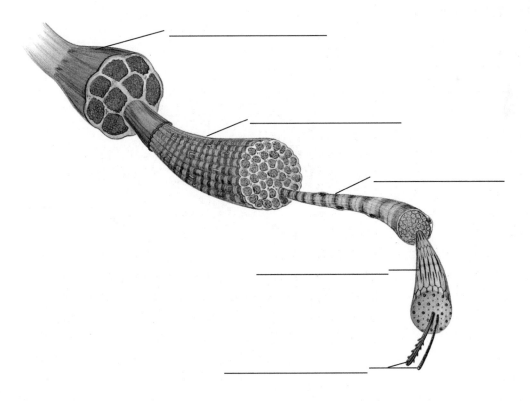

_____

_____

_____

_____

_____

13. Figure 8-19

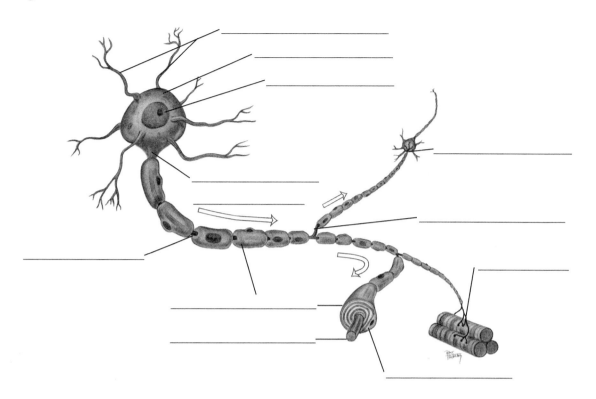

Chapter 9: Oral Mucosa

14. Figure 9-1

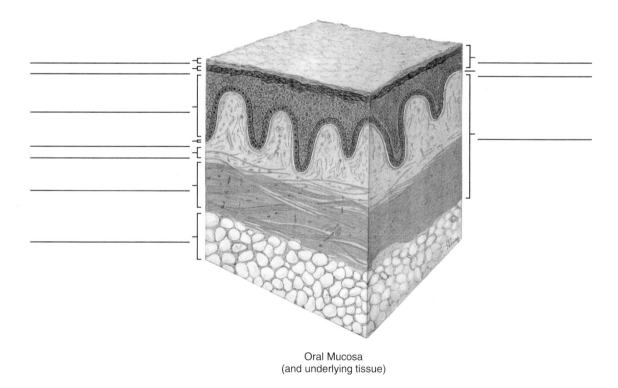

Oral Mucosa
(and underlying tissue)

15. Figure 9-2

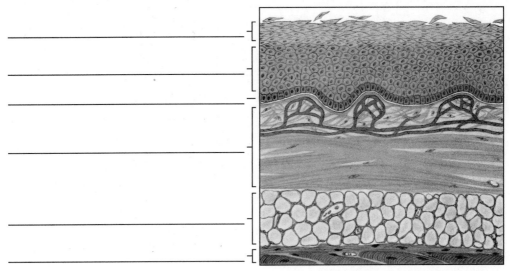

Nonkeratinized Stratified Squamous Epithelium
(and deeper tissue)

16. Figure 9-3

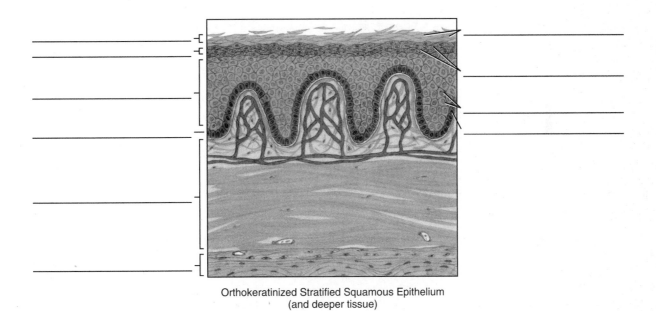

Orthokeratinized Stratified Squamous Epithelium
(and deeper tissue)

17. Figure 9-5

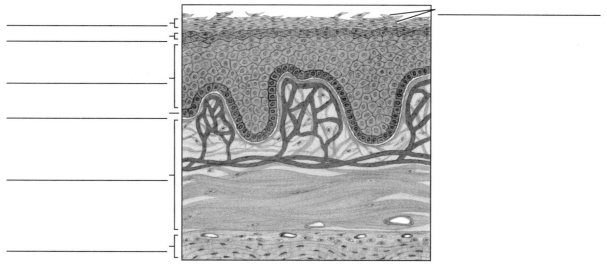

Parakeratinized Stratified Squamous Epithelium
(and deeper tissue)

18. Figure 9-6

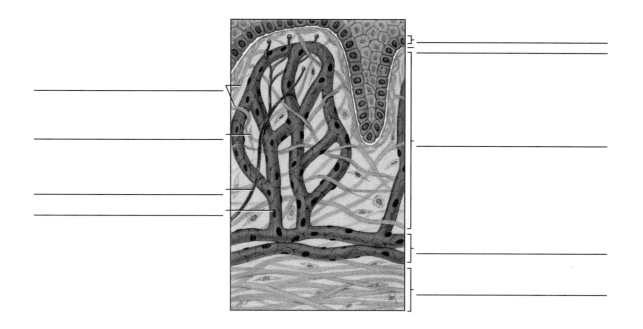

19.   Figure 9-13

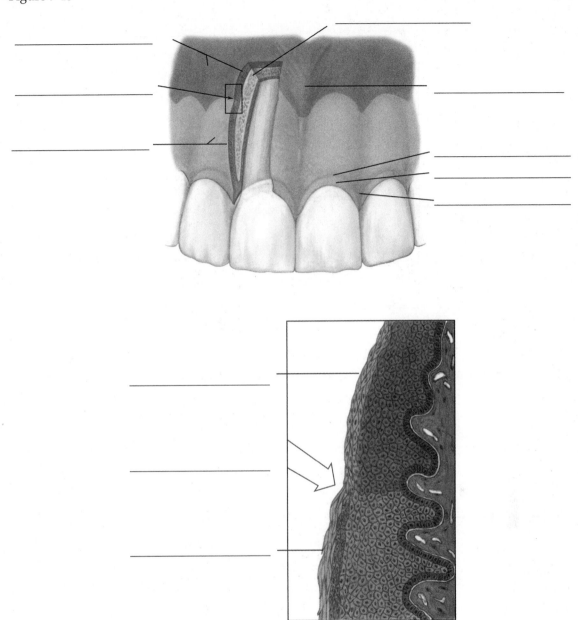

20. Figure 9-17

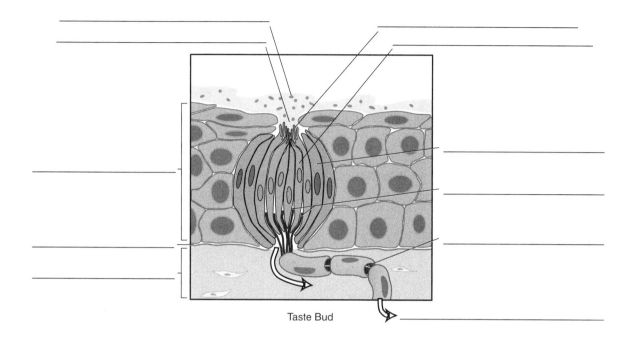

Taste Bud

Chapter 10: Gingival and Dentogingival Junctional Tissue

21. Figure 10-1

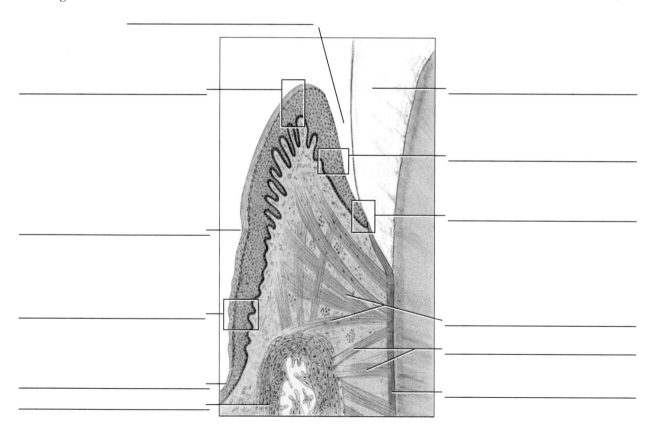

22. Figure 10-6

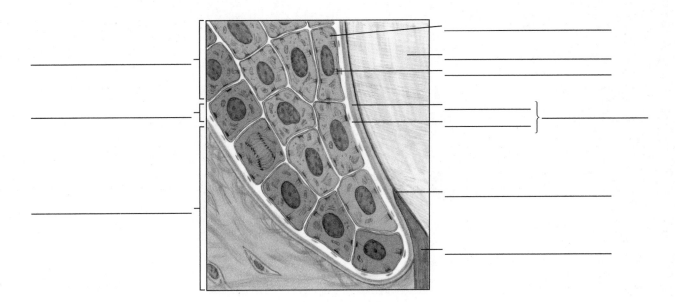

Chapter 11: Head and Neck Structures

23. Figure 11-1, *B*

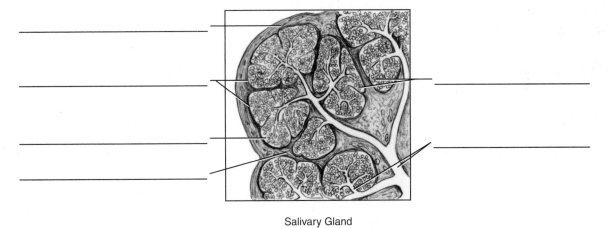

Salivary Gland

24. Figure 11-6

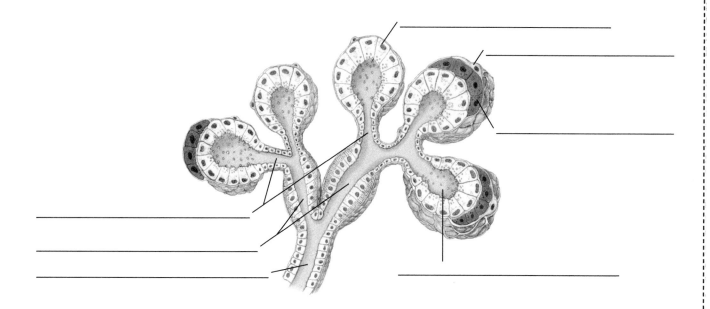

25. Figure 11-7, *A, B, C*

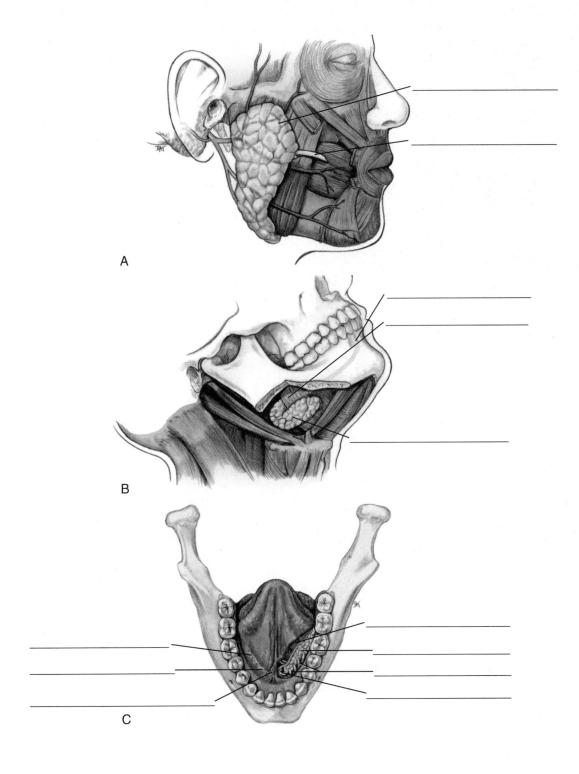

A

B

C

26. Figure 11-13, *B*

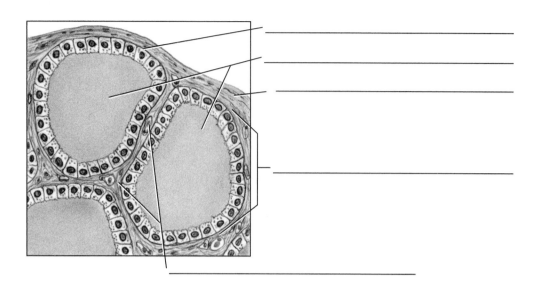

27. Figure 11-16, *A*

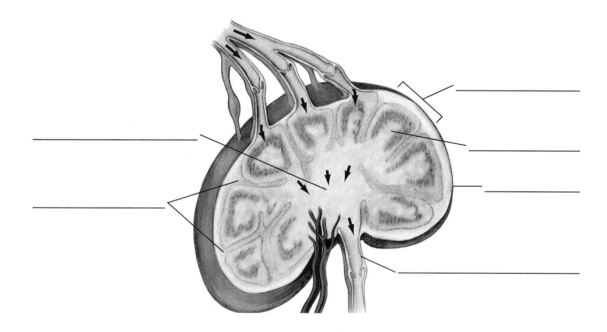

28.   Figure 11-17, *A*

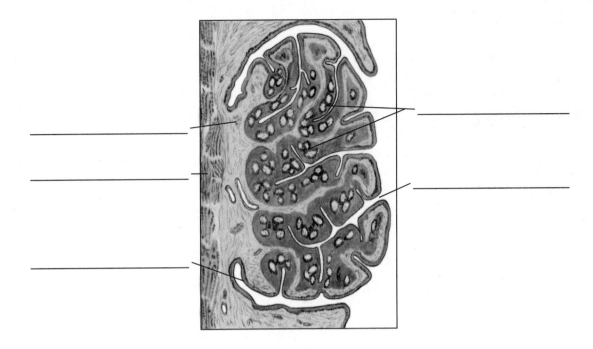

29.   Figure 11-19

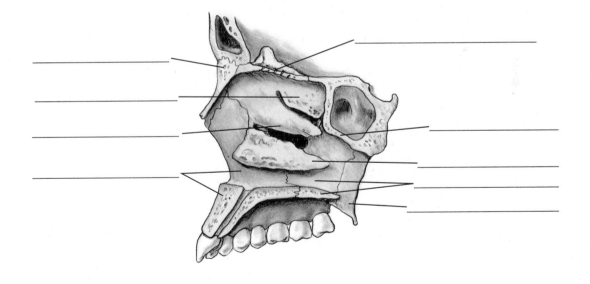

30. Figure 11-20

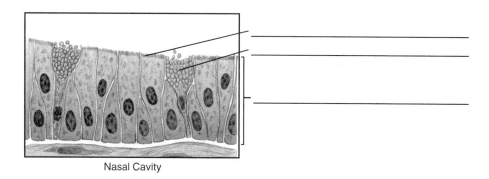

Nasal Cavity

31. Figure 11-21

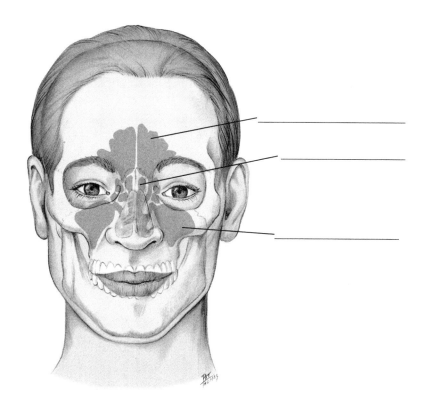

Chapter 12: Enamel

32. Figure 12-4, *A* and *B*, Figure 12-6, *A*

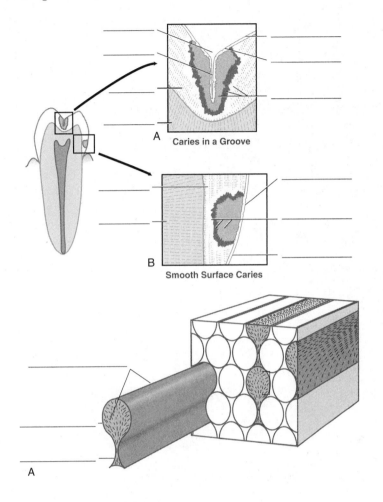

A   Caries in a Groove

B   Smooth Surface Caries

A

Chapter 13: Dentin and Pulp

33. Figure 13-9, Figure 13-16

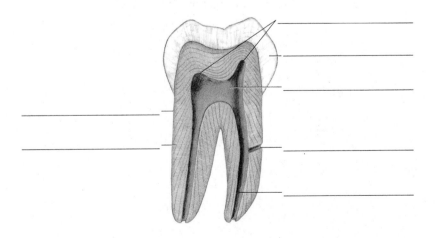

Chapter 14: Periodontium: Cementum, Alveolar Process, and Periodontal Ligament

34.   Figure 14-1

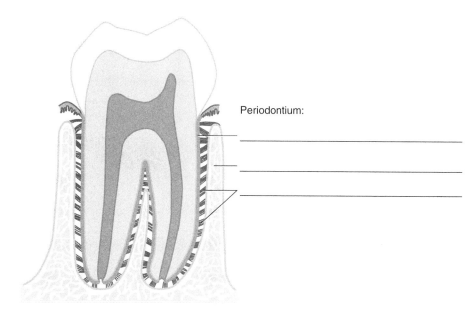

Periodontium:

35.   Figure 14-2

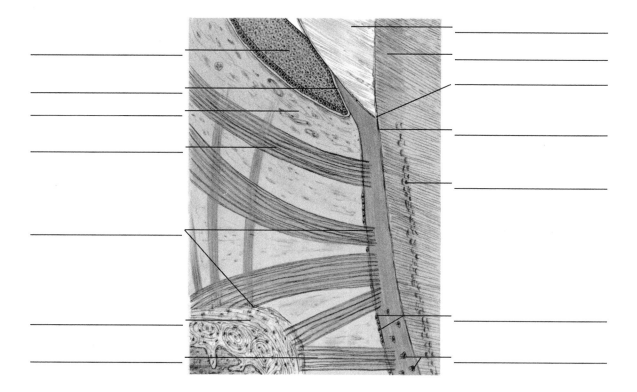

36. Figure 14-14, *A, B, C* (Courtesy of Margaret J. Fehrenbach, RDH, MS.)

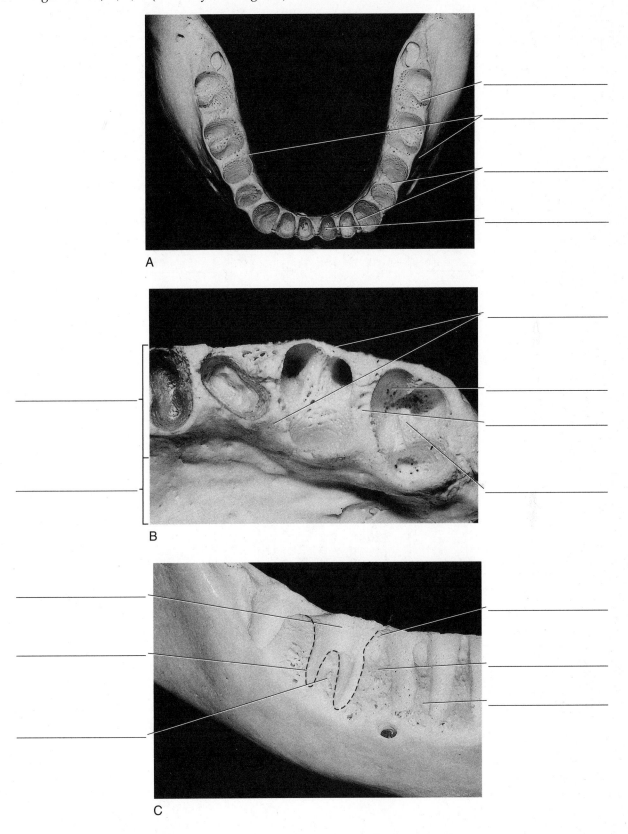

37. Figure 14-20

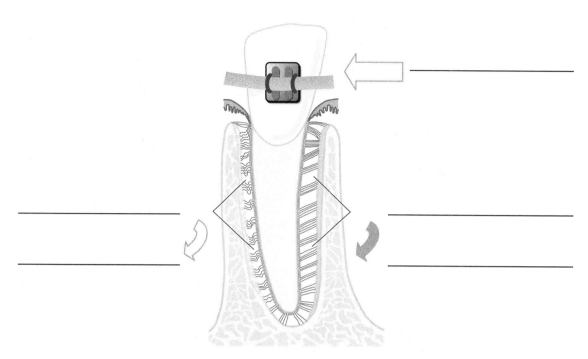

Orthodontic Tooth Movement

38. Figure 14-27

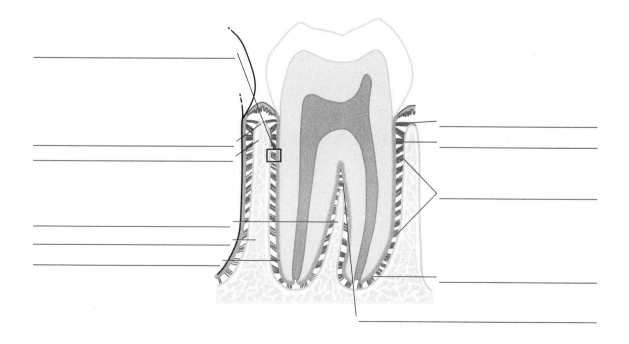

39. Figure 14-31

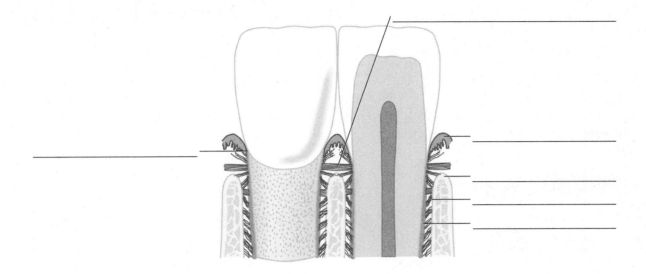

40. Figure 14-32

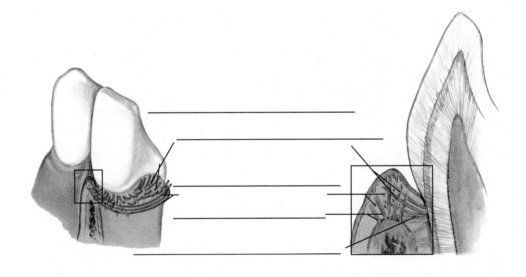

UNIT IV: DENTAL ANATOMY

Chapter 15: Overview of Dentitions

1. Figure 15-1

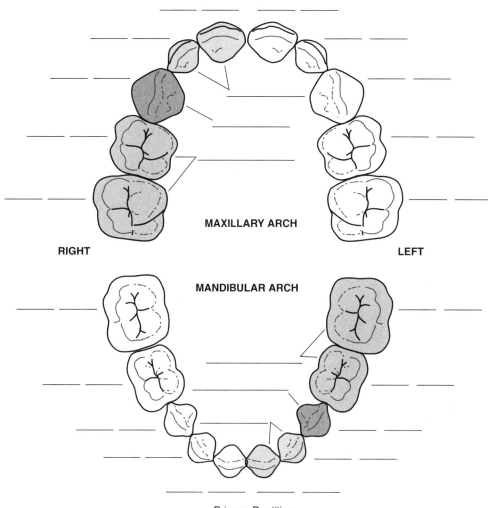

MAXILLARY ARCH

RIGHT   LEFT

MANDIBULAR ARCH

Primary Dentition

2. Figure 15-2

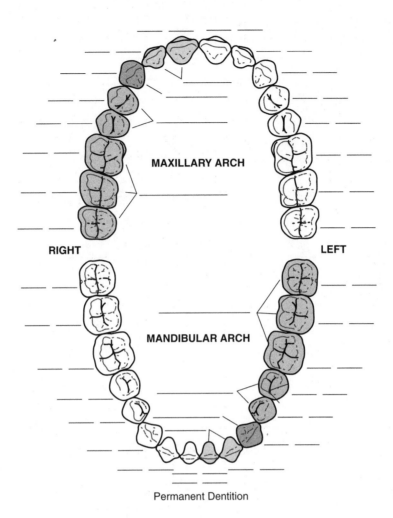

MAXILLARY ARCH

RIGHT   LEFT

MANDIBULAR ARCH

Permanent Dentition

3. Figure 15-5

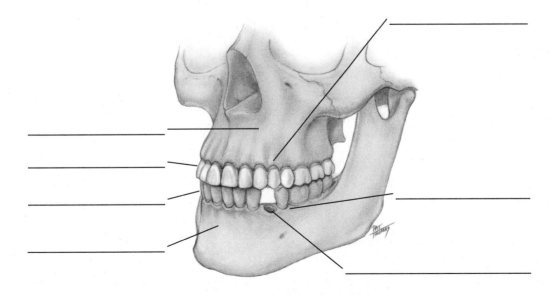

4. Figure 15-6

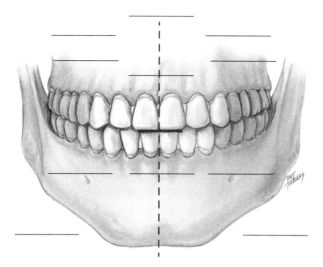

5. Figure 15-7

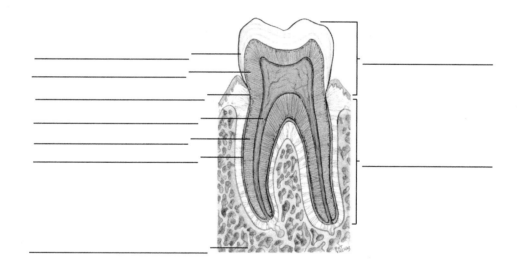

6.   Figure 15-8

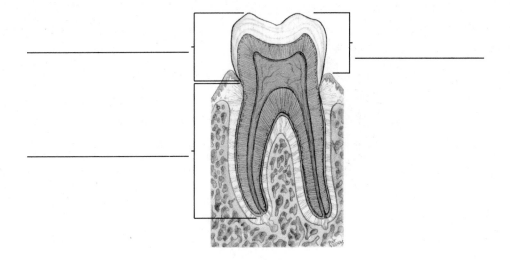

7.   Figure 15-9

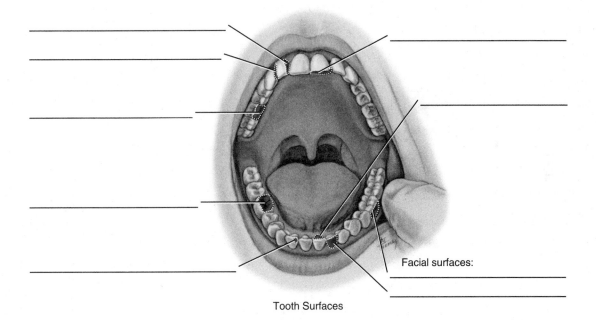

Facial surfaces:

Tooth Surfaces

8. Figure 15-11

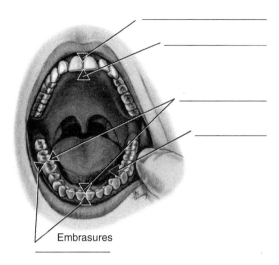

Embrasures

9. Figure 15-12

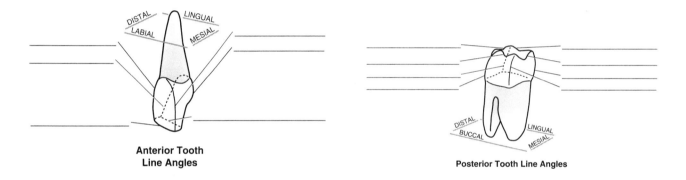

**Anterior Tooth
Line Angles**

Posterior Tooth Line Angles

10. Figure 15-14

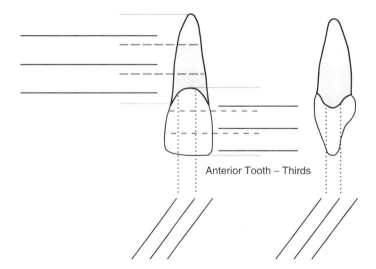

Anterior Tooth – Thirds

11. Figure 15-14 (continued)

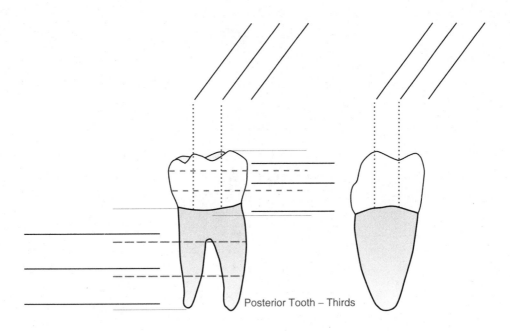

Posterior Tooth – Thirds

Chapter 16: Permanent Anterior Teeth

12. Figure 16-7

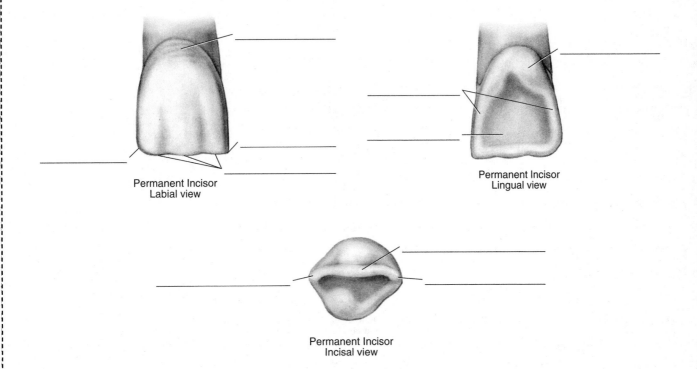

Permanent Incisor
Labial view

Permanent Incisor
Lingual view

Permanent Incisor
Incisal view

13. Figure 16-16

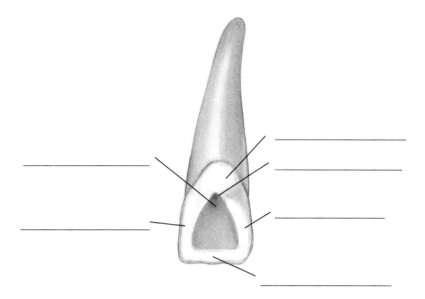

Permanent Maxillary Right Lateral Incisor
Lingual View

14. Figure 16-22

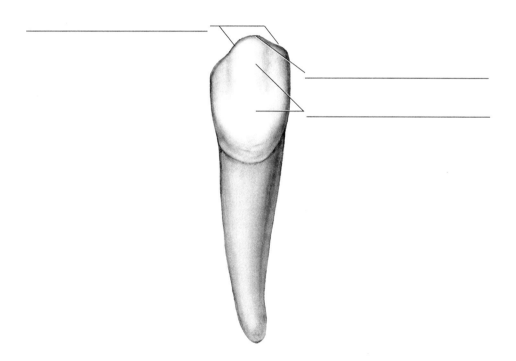

Permanent Mandibular Right Canine
Labial View

15. Figure 16-23

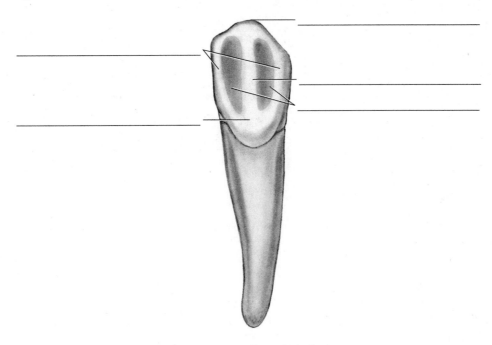

Permanent Mandibular Right Canine
Lingual View

16. Figure 16-27

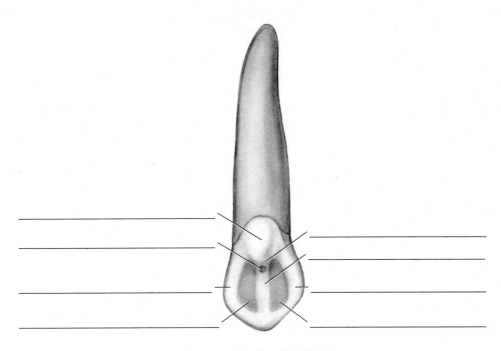

Permanent Maxillary Right Canine
Lingual View

Chapter 17: Permanent Posterior Teeth

17.   Figure 17-2

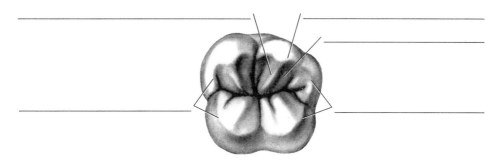

Permanent Posterior Tooth
Occlusal View

18.   Figure 17-4

Developmental Grooves:

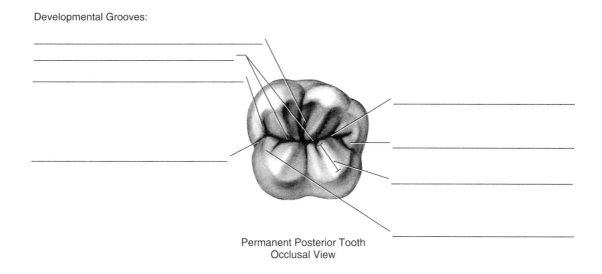

Permanent Posterior Tooth
Occlusal View

19.   Figure 17-7

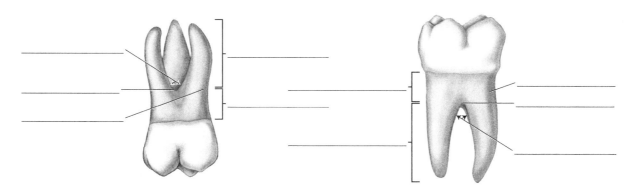

Permanent Posterior Molars: Maxillary and Mandibular
Buccal Views

20.   Figure 17-10

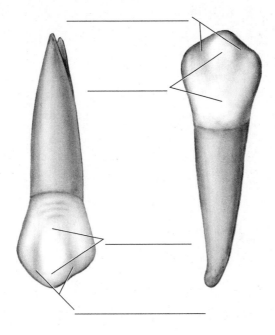

Permanent Premolars
Buccal Views

21.   Figure 17-13

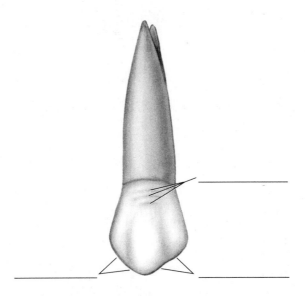

Permanent Maxillary Right First Premolar
Buccal View

22. Figure 17-14

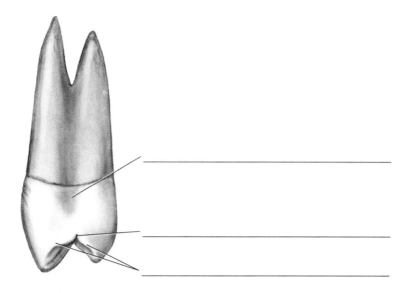

Permanent Maxillary Right First Premolar
Mesial View

23. Figure 17-15

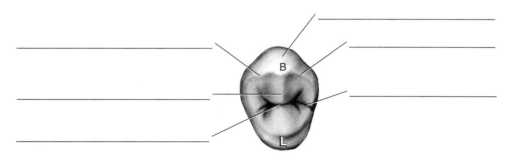

Permanent Maxillary Right First Premolar
Occlusal View

24. Figure 17-16

Transverse {
Ridge {

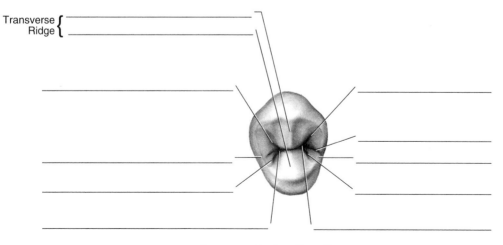

Permanent Maxillary Right First Premolar
Occlusal View

25.   Figure 17-19

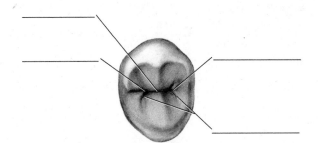

Permanent Maxillary Right Second Premolar
Occlusal View

26.   Figure 17-22

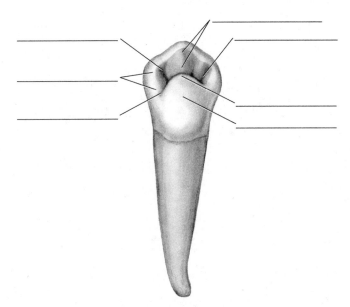

Permanent Mandibular Right First Premolar
Lingual View

27.   Figure 17-23

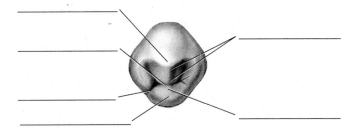

Permanent Mandibular Right First Premolar
Occlusal View

28. Figure 17-24

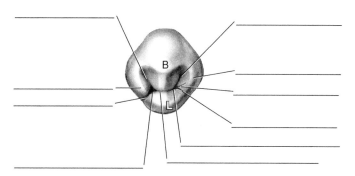

Permanent Mandibular Right First Premolar
Occlusal View

29. Figure 17-27

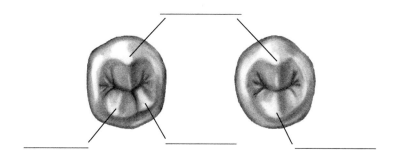

Three-Cusp type   **Two-Cusp type**

Permanent Mandibular Second Premolars
Occlusal Views

30. Figure 17-29

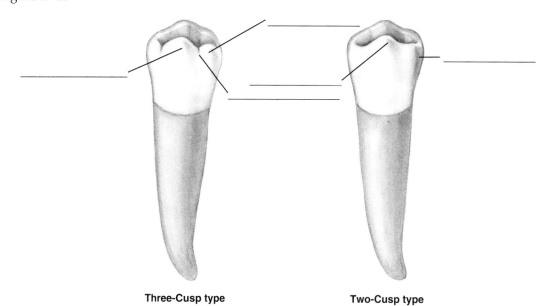

Three-Cusp type   **Two-Cusp type**

Permanent Mandibular Right First Premolars
Lingual Views

31. Figure 17-30

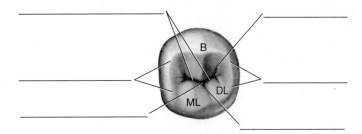

Permanent Mandibular Right Second Premolar: Three-Cusp Type, Y-Shaped Groove Pattern
Occlusal View

32. Figure 17-31

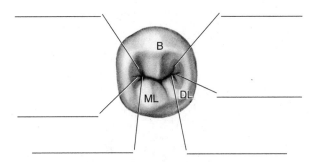

Permanent Mandibular Right Second Premolar: Three-Cusp Type
Occlusal View

33. Figure 17-32

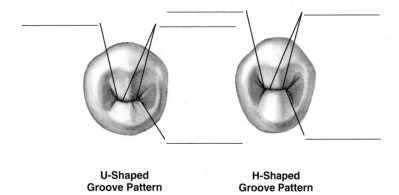

**U-Shaped
Groove Pattern**   **H-Shaped
Groove Pattern**

Permanent Mandibular Right Second Premolars: Two-Cusp Type
Occlusal View

34. Figure 17-34

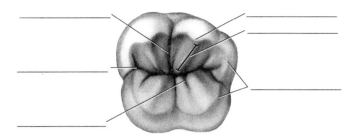

Permanent Molar
Occlusal View

35. Figure 17-37

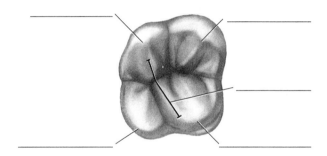

Permanent Maxillary Molar
Occlusal View

36. Figure 17-41

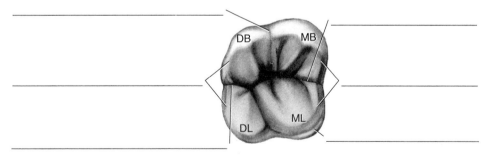

Permanent Maxillary Right First Molar
Occlusal View

37. Figure 17-42

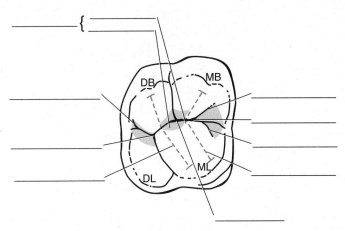

Permanent Maxillary Right First Molar
Occlusal View

38. Figure 17-46

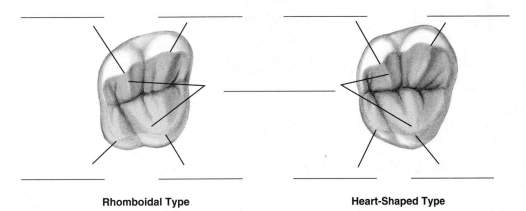

Rhomboidal Type   **Heart-Shaped Type**

Permanent Maxillary Right Second Molars
Occlusal Views

39. Figure 17-53

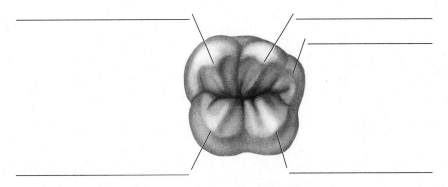

Permanent Mandibular Right First Molar
Occlusal View

40. Figure 17-54

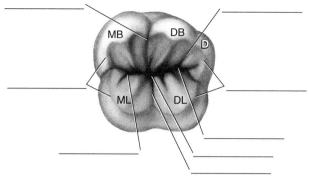

Permanent Maxillary Right First Molar
Occlusal View

41. Figure 17-59

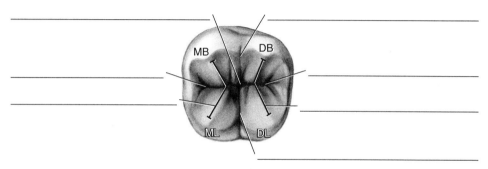

Permanent Mandibular Right Second Molar
Occlusal View

Chapter 18: Primary Dentition

42. Figure 18-2

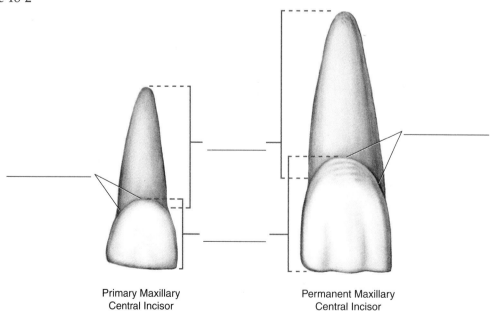

Primary Maxillary
Central Incisor

Permanent Maxillary
Central Incisor

Labial Views

43. Figure 18-3

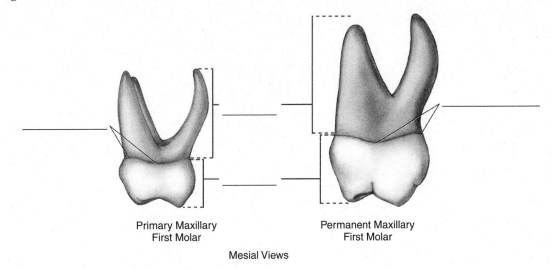

Primary Maxillary
First Molar

Permanent Maxillary
First Molar

Mesial Views

Chapter 19: Temporomandibular Joint

44. Figure 19-1

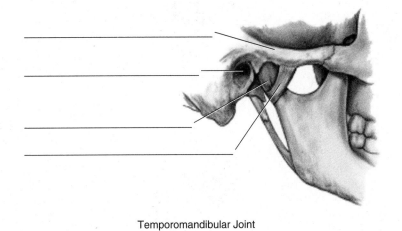

Temporomandibular Joint

45. Figure 19-5

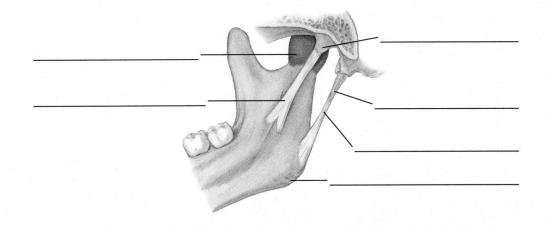

46. Figure 19-6

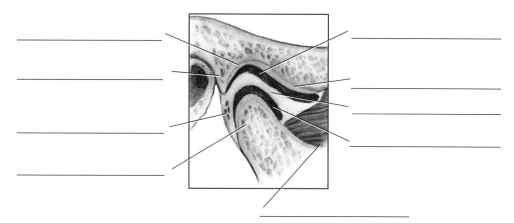

47. Figure 19-8, *A, B, C*

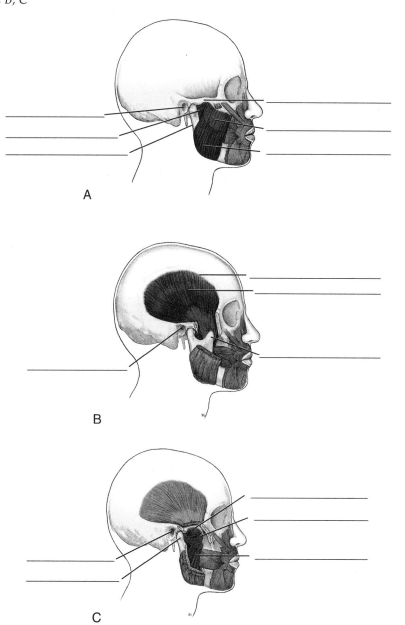

A

B

C

Basic Clinical Supplies Needed: The student dental professional will need the following basic supplies for the clinical identification exercises: dental chair and light, mirror instrument, hand mirror, and workbook-included checklist. Standard infection control precautions, including personal protection equipment, must be adhered to as outlined by the Occupational Safety and Health Administration Bloodborne Pathogens Standard (see reference in Infection Control Procedures for Extracted Teeth). Both Universal and International Numbering Systems are included in the checklists.

After completing the medical and dental history and review, the patient should be seated in a dental chair, either supine or upright as needed. Use preprocedural antimicrobial mouthrinse, remove any pigmented lipsticks, and apply non-petroleum lubricant to dry lips; ask to take out any removable prostheses. Good lighting and exposure of the area being assessed are essential (e.g., collar and tie loosened, glasses removed).

Explanations of the reasons for performing extraoral and intraoral examinations as well as examination of the dentition and occlusion and their relationship of these examinations to dental treatment, including the terms used in these examinations, are located in the associated textbook in **Chapters 1, 2, 15, and 20.** More in-depth examination of these areas can be done in the future by student dental professionals after additional coursework in oral pathology, periodontology, dental materials, radiology, and clinical rotations.

Part 1: CLINICAL IDENTIFICATION EXERCISE: Extraoral Structures

Directions: During this exercise in extraoral structure identification, check the items as noted. Use both visual inspection and palpation during the examination, making sure to also note any variations such as with traumatic injury, if applicable. Include specific location using nearby structures. Also note any atypical findings; if found, take non-identifiable clinical photographs to be shared (after being granted permission) with other students, and make appropriate referrals. Include also any palpable lymph nodes of the face and neck, if applicable.

Regions of the Face Checklist		
Frontal, Orbital, and Nasal Regions	**Variations**	**Atypical Findings**
Forehead		
Orbits		
External Nose: Root of Nose, Apex of Nose, Nares, Nasal Septum, Nasal Alae		
Infraorbital Zygomatic Regions	**Variations**	**Atypical Findings**
Zygomatic Arches		
Temporomandibular Joints		
Buccal Regions	**Variations**	**Atypical Findings**
Cheeks and Masseter Muscles		
Angles of the Mandible		
Parotid Salivary Glands		
Oral Region	**Variations**	**Atypical Findings**
Lips: Vermilion Zone, Mucocutaneous Junction, Labial Commissures		
Maxilla, Philtrum, Tubercle of Upper Lip		
Mental Region	**Variations**	**Atypical Findings**
Mandible: Mandibular Symphysis, Rami, Coronoid Processes, Coronoid Notches, Mandibular Condyles, Mandibular Notches		

Regions of the Neck	Variations	Atypical Findings
Sternocleidomastoid muscles		
Hyoid Bone		
Thyroid Cartilage		
Thyroid Gland		
Submandibular Salivary Glands		
Sublingual Salivary Glands		

Part 2: CLINICAL IDENTIFICATION EXERCISE: Intraoral Structures

Directions: During this exercise in intraoral structure identification, check the items as noted. Use both visual inspection and palpation during the examination, making sure to also note any variations such as Fordyce spots, linea alba, exostoses, mandibular tori, and palatal torus, if applicable. Include specific location using nearby structures. Also note any atypical findings; if found, take non-identifiable clinical photographs to be shared (after being granted permission) with other students, and make appropriate referrals.

The posterior part of the base of the tongue and its structures, such as the lingual tonsil, are usually not visible when examining the oral cavity; however, note the relationship of the nasopharynx and laryngopharynx to the oropharynx by indicating on the external neck the placement of these related internal regions. When examining oral mucosal surfaces, it is important to gently dry those surfaces with a gauze or air syringe, so that color or texture changes will become more obvious. In addition, avoid palpation of any structures near the soft palate or pharynx to prevent the gag reflex; use only visual inspection in this area.

Oral Cavity Checklist		
Oral Vestibules	**Variations**	**Atypical Findings**
Labial Mucosa		
Buccal Mucosa, Buccal Fat Pads		
Parotid Salivary Glands, Parotid Papillae		
Vestibular Fornix		
Alveolar Mucosa, Mucobuccal Fold		
Labial Frena: Maxillary and Mandibular		
Jaws, Alveolar Processes, Teeth, Arches	**Variations**	**Atypical Findings**
Maxilla: Body, Maxillary Sinuses, Alveolar Process, Alveoli, Canine Eminences, Maxillary Teeth, Maxillary Tuberosities		
Mandible: Body, Alveolar Process, Alveoli, Canine Eminences, Mandibular Teeth, Retromolar Pads		
Permanent Teeth within Maxillary and Mandibular Arches: Crown, Enamel, Anterior Teeth (Incisors, Canines), Posterior Teeth (Premolars, and Molars)		

Gingival Tissue	Variations	Atypical Findings
Attached Gingiva		
Mucogingival Junction		
Marginal Gingiva: Free Gingival Crest and Groove		
Gingival Sulci (location only)		
Interdental Gingiva: Interdental Papillae		
Oral Cavity Proper	**Variations**	**Atypical Findings**
Fauces: Anterior and Posterior Pillars		
Palatine Tonsils		
Palate	**Variations**	**Atypical Findings**
Hard Palate: Median Palatine Raphe, Incisive Papilla, Palatine Rugae		
Soft Palate, Uvula		
Pterygomandibular Folds		
Tongue	**Variations**	**Atypical Findings**
Base of Tongue (anterior part only)		
Body of Tongue		
Dorsal Surface: Median Lingual Sulcus, Sulcus Terminalis, Foramen Cecum (if possible)		
Filiform Lingual Papillae		
Circumvallate Lingual Papillae		
Lateral Surfaces		
Foliate Lingual Papillae		
Ventral Surface		
Plicae Fimbriatae		
Floor of the Mouth	**Variations**	**Atypical Findings**
Lingual Frenum		
Sublingual Folds		
Sublingual Caruncles		
Sublingual Salivary Glands		
Submandibular Salivary Glands		
Pharynx	**Variations**	**Atypical Findings**
Oropharynx		

Part 3: CLINICAL IDENTIFICATION EXERCISE: Tooth Types in Permanent Dentition

Directions: During this exercise in identifying tooth types in the permanent dentition, circle the items as noted on the crowns of the tooth types listed. Place **NA (Not Applicable)** if trauma, restoration, or extraction has occurred to the tooth crown so that it is impossible to tell what is present; third molars will not be specifically examined, but take notes on crown anatomy, if present. Compare both sides of each arch when investigating; the sequence below is the same as the one used for discussion in the associated textbook. Use both the instrument mirror and explorer during the examination, making sure to also note any variations or atypical findings; if found, take non-identifiable clinical photographs to be shared (after being granted permission) with other students, and make appropriate referrals.

INCISORS CHECKLIST

TOOTH NUMBER	INCISAL SURFACE	CINGULUM/ MARGINAL RIDGES	LINGUAL FOSSA	NOTES
8, 9 (11, 21)	Ridge/Edge	Well developed/ Not noticeable	Deep/Shallow	
7, 10 (12, 22)	Ridge/Edge	Well developed/ Not noticeable	Deep/Shallow	
24, 25 (31, 41)	Ridge/Edge	Well developed/ Not noticeable	Deep/Shallow	
23, 26 (32, 42)	Ridge/Edge	Well developed/ Not noticeable	Deep/Shallow	

CANINES CHECKLIST

TOOTH NUMBER	CUSP TIP	CINGULUM/ LINGUAL RIDGE/ MARGINAL RIDGES	LINGUAL FOSSA	NOTES
6, 11 (13, 23)	Centered/ Offset	Well developed/ Not noticeable	Deep/Shallow	
22, 27 (33, 43)	Centered/ Offset	Well developed/ Not noticeable	Deep/Shallow	

PREMOLARS CHECKLIST

TOOTH NUMBER	OCCLUSAL SHAPE	CUSPS	RIDGES	PROXIMAL SHAPE	NOTES
5, 12 (14, 24)	Hexagon/Diamond-Shaped/Square	2 or 3	Transverse/ Not Transverse	Trapezoid/ Rhomboid	
4, 13 (15, 25)	Hexagon/Diamond-Shaped/Square	2 or 3	Transverse/Not Transverse	Trapezoid/ Rhomboid	
21, 28 (34, 44)	Hexagon/Diamond-Shaped/Square	2 or 3	Transverse/Not Transverse	Trapezoid/ Rhomboid	
20, 29 (35, 45)	Hexagon/Diamond-Shaped/Square	2 or 3	Transverse/Not Transverse	Trapezoid/ Rhomboid	

MOLARS CHECKLIST

TOOTH NUMBER	OCCLUSAL SHAPE	CUSPS	RIDGES	PROXIMAL SHAPE	PITS	NOTES
3, 14 (16, 26)	Rhomboid/ Heart-Shaped	4 or 5	Oblique/ Transverse	Trapezoid/ Rhomboid	Lingual/ Buccal	
2, 15 (17, 27)	Rhomboid/ Heart-Shaped	4 or 5	Oblique/ Transverse	Trapezoid/ Rhomboid	Lingual/ Buccal	
19, 30 (36, 46)	Rectang/ Pentagon	4 or 5	Oblique/ Transverse	Trapezoid/ Rhomboid	Lingual/ Buccal	
18, 31 (37, 47)	Rectang/ Pentagon	4 or 5	Oblique/ Transverse	Trapezoid/ Rhomboid	Lingual/ Buccal	
1, 16 (18, 28)						
17, 32 (38, 48)						

Part 4: CLINICAL IDENTIFICATION EXERCISE: Permanent Occlusion

Additional Supplies Needed: The student dental professional will need the following additional supplies during these exercises for the clinical identification of an occlusion of a permanent dentition: periodontal probe instrument, articulating paper, and floss. Many steps are involved in this procedure but the sequence executed can be modified as needed; the sequence below is the same as the one used for discussion in the associated textbook. If there are interesting features to the occlusion, take non-identifiable clinical photographs to be shared (after being granted permission) with the other students, and make appropriate referrals.

Step 1. Occlusal History with Extraoral and Intraoral Findings

Before performing the identification of an occlusion, take notes on the **occlusal history** of the patient. Note in the chart any removable prostheses (flippers, retainers, night and sports mouthguards, and partial and/or complete dentures), and have the patient keep them in during the procedure if worn regularly. Record any occlusal complaints, habits, and applicable physical or psychological findings from the patient or medical history questionnaire that may be pertinent to the patient's occlusal history. Note these findings under occlusal history.

Additionally, note any information found during an **extraoral examination** that may be pertinent to the patient's occlusion (see earlier discussion). This includes the facial profile and any asymmetries, loss of vertical dimension, mandibular deviation upon opening, and temporomandibular disorder signs. Also note any information found during an intraoral examination that may be pertinent to the patient's occlusion. Note the general amount of **attrition** or **abfraction** of the dentition, and record the location and amount of associated wear facets or cervical lesions involved in the area provided on the chart. Finally, note any **mobility** of the dentition by circling the involved teeth in red opposite the mobility section.

Record any **sensitivity** to thermal changes or percussion (gentle tapping). Record any deviations in the **intra-arch form or alignment**, such as loss of contact, plunging cusps, open bite, crossbites, and any arch collapse. Note also any missing, rotated, supererupted, drifted, or fractured teeth, or those with abfraction. Include any changes in restorations; occlusal trauma is the main reason for early restoration failure. Changes in the midline of the two dentitions should also be noted. Note these items related to intra-arch findings in the areas listed on the chart.

Finally, record any pertinent information from a **radiographic examination** of the dentition, if available, such as amount of bone support, alterations of the periodontal ligament, root resorption, nonvital and fixed prosthetic teeth, including veneers, crowns, and implants. Record these findings in the area listed as the radiographic examination.

Step 2. Achieving Centric Relation Through Patient-Clinician

To allow the student dental professional to identify the occlusion of a patient, the patient must be first in Centric Relation (CR). The position of **CR** is the end point of closure of the mandible in which the mandible is in the most retruded position, which will serve as a baseline for an occlusal evaluation.

To achieve CR, first place the patient in an upright position, sitting or standing in front and to the side of the patient. The patient should be relaxed, looking straight ahead with lips parted. Using the operating hand, place a thumb against the outside of the patient's chin, with the fingers placed under the inferior border of the mandible to alternately lift and loosen the mandible. Then, establish the hinge movement of the mandible by gently arcing the mandible with the fingers several times in a closing and opening manner. Then, guide the loosened mandible into closure, with the mandible placed in its most retruded position.

Step 3. Determining Angle Classification of Malocclusion

Once the patient is in CR, determine the **angle classification of malocclusion** of the patient's dentition. Most cases can be placed into one of three main classes on the basis of the position of the permanent maxillary first molar relative to the mandibular first molar (see text). The position of the canines in each arch must also be noted if the first molars cannot be used for classification. A tendency to any type of malocclusion, which is considered less than the width of a premolar, can be noted using either the molar or canine relationship. Additionally, any subgroups within the classification must be noted as well if the right or left side are not symmetrical in classification. The classification is recorded in the area on the chart labeled "Angle classification."

Step 4. Measuring Overjet

With the patient maintained in CR, **overjet,** or horizontal overlap between the two arches, is determined by measuring it in millimeters with the tip of the periodontal probe. Place the probe at a right angle to the labial surface of a mandibular incisor at the base of the incisal ridge of a maxillary incisor. The measurement is taken from the labial surface of the mandibular incisor to the lingual surface of the maxillary incisor. Note that the labiolingual width of the maxillary incisor is not included in the measurement. The overjet measurement is recorded in the chart in the area labeled "Overjet."

Step 5. Measuring Overbite

Overbite, or vertical overlap between the two arches, is determined also by measuring it in millimeters with the tip of the periodontal probe after the patient is placed in CR. Place the probe on the incisal ridge of the maxillary incisor at right angle to the mandibular incisor. As the patient opens the mouth or depresses the jaws, then place the probe vertically against the mandibular incisor to measure the distance to the incisal ridge of the mandibular incisor. The overbite measurement is recorded in the chart in the area labeled "Overbite."

Step 6. Checking for Interocclusal Clearance

Allow the patient to rest while checking for **interocclusal clearance**, the space when the mandible is at rest. In this rest position, an average space of 2 to 3 mm can be noted between the masticatory surfaces of the maxillary and mandibular teeth. Thus, failure of a patient to assume this position when the jaws are not at work may mean the patient is habitually tense or has parafunctional habits such as clenching or grinding (bruxism). Interocclusal clearance is measured in millimeters and recorded in that area on the chart. If there is no interocclusal clearance noted during mandibular rest, follow-up questions may be necessary to ascertain any habitual tension or parafunctional habits.

Step 7. Checking for Premature Contact

After the patient relaxes for a moment, the position of CR can again be attained, and the patient is then asked where the teeth first touch during occlusion by having them close their teeth gently together. If it is a single tooth, the tooth is considered to be a **premature contact**. Articulation paper can then be used to check for these premature contacts, which limit the opportunity for maximal intercuspation of the teeth. Premature contacts are recorded in the chart by circling the tooth numbers of the contacting teeth in red opposite the CR occlusion section.

Step 8. Achieving Centric Occlusion

Next, have the patient clench the teeth together, and note the amount of shift in millimeters from jaw position in CR to jaw position in Centric Occlusion (CO), as well as its direction. **CO**, or habitual occlusion, is the voluntary position of the dentition that allows maximal contact when the teeth occlude. Record the amount of shift in millimeters in the chart; record also the direction of the shift (anterior, right, left, posterior). Ideally, no shift is noted since the position of the teeth in CR is the same as in CO, and CR = CO is circled in the chart. However, the average distance of shift from a patient's occlusion in CR to CO is approximately 1 mm or less, in an anterior to posterior direction.

Step 9. Checking Lateral Occlusion

Next, it is necessary to check the patient's occlusion within lateral deviation or excursion. **Lateral occlusion** is evaluated by moving the mandible to either the right or the left until the canines on that side are in **canine rise**, or cuspid rise. The patient's mandible is supported with the operating hand, and then the mandible is gently moved into CR or even CO. Then, slowly guide the mandible to the patient's right or left until the opposing canines are edge-to-edge.

The side to which the mandible has been moved is the **working side**. There are two working sides noted in an occlusal evaluation: right lateral and left lateral. Before the opposing canines come into contact on each side, other individual teeth that make contact on the working side should be noted. These **working contacts** are recorded by circling the tooth numbers of the contacting teeth in blue on the chart in the area opposite the lateral occlusion section for the appropriate side.

The side of the arch that is opposite or contralateral to the working side during lateral occlusion is the **balancing side** or **nonworking side**. If any teeth make contact on the balancing side during lateral occlusion, they are recorded as a **balancing interference** and are circled in red for the appropriate side. If **group function** is present, most of the entire posterior quadrant of each arch is functioning during lateral occlusion without canine rise. This should be recorded by circling the tooth numbers of the involved group of teeth in blue on the chart opposite the lateral occlusion section for the appropriate side.

Do not allow patients to move freely into lateral deviation, because they may choose a convenient path to bypass a balancing interference within the occlusion. For further confirmation of any balancing interferences during lateral deviation, place floss across the retromolar pads extending out to the labial commissures, or place articulating paper over the occlusal surfaces on the appropriate side. After guiding the patient into either right or left lateral occlusion, slip the floss or articulating paper forward, noting any points of contact.

Step 10. Checking Protrusive Occlusion

Finally, check the **protrusive occlusion** of the patient. With the patient's teeth in CO, support the mandible with the operating hand and have the patient slowly move the mandible forward so that the two dentitions are in an edge-to-edge relationship. Note any posterior tooth or canine contacts as well as **balancing interferences** during protrusion, and record this information on the chart by circling the contacting teeth in red opposite the protrusive section. Also note the anterior teeth that are in contact during protrusion, or the **working contacts,** by circling on the chart the tooth numbers of the contacting teeth in blue opposite the protrusive section.

For further confirmation of working contacts and any balancing interferences during protrusion, place the floss across the retromolar pads extending out to the labial commissures. Then, guide the patient into protrusive occlusion, and slip the floss forward between the teeth until resistance of contacting teeth is met.

OCCLUSAL IDENTIFICATION FORM

Occlusal History _____

_____

Extraoral Findings _____

_____

Intraoral Findings _____

_____

Angle Classification _____ **Right** _____ **Left** _____ **Subgroup** _____

Molar Right _____ **Canine Right** _____ **Molar Left** _____ **Canine Left** _____

Interocclusal Clearance _____ **mm Sensitivity** _____

Overjet _____ **mm Overbite** _____ **mm Attrition** _____ **Abfraction** _____

Intra-Arch Form/Alignment _____

_____

Radiographic Examination (if available) _____

_____

OCCLUSAL IDENTIFICATION CHECKLIST

Centric Relation **Centric Occlusion**	1 2 3 4 5 6 7 8 (18 17 16 15 14 13 12 11)	9 10 11 12 13 14 15 16 (21 22 23 24 25 26 27 28)
	32 31 30 29 28 27 26 25 (48 47 46 45 44 43 42 41)	24 23 22 21 20 19 18 17 (31 32 33 34 35 36 37 38)
CR = CO	**Shift CR to CO ____ mm**	**Anterior Right Left Posterior**
Right Lateral **Occlusion**	1 2 3 4 5 6 7 8 (18 17 16 15 14 13 12 11)	9 10 11 12 13 14 15 16 (21 22 23 24 25 26 27 28)
	32 31 30 29 28 27 26 25 (48 47 46 45 44 43 42 41)	24 23 22 21 20 19 18 17 (31 32 33 34 35 36 37 38)
Left Lateral **Occlusion**	1 2 3 4 5 6 7 8 (18 17 16 15 14 13 12 11)	9 10 11 12 13 14 15 16 (21 22 23 24 25 26 27 28)
	32 31 30 29 28 27 26 25 (48 47 46 45 44 43 42 41)	24 23 22 21 20 19 18 17 (31 32 33 34 35 36 37 38)
Protrusive **Occlusion**	1 2 3 4 5 6 7 8 (18 17 16 15 14 13 12 11)	9 10 11 12 13 14 15 16 (21 22 23 24 25 26 27 28)
	32 31 30 29 28 27 26 25 (48 47 46 45 44 43 42 41)	24 23 22 21 20 19 18 17 (31 32 33 34 35 36 37 38)
Wear Facets	1 2 3 4 5 6 7 8 (18 17 16 15 14 13 12 11)	9 10 11 12 13 14 15 16 (21 22 23 24 25 26 27 28)
	32 31 30 29 28 27 26 25 (48 47 46 45 44 43 42 41)	24 23 22 21 20 19 18 17 (31 32 33 34 35 36 37 38)
Cervical Lesions	1 2 3 4 5 6 7 8 (18 17 16 15 14 13 12 11)	9 10 11 12 13 14 15 16 (21 22 23 24 25 26 27 28)
	32 31 30 29 28 27 26 25 (48 47 46 45 44 43 42 41)	24 23 22 21 20 19 18 17 (31 32 33 34 35 36 37 38)
Mobility	1 2 3 4 5 6 7 8 (18 17 16 15 14 13 12 11)	9 10 11 12 13 14 15 16 (21 22 23 24 25 26 27 28)
	32 31 30 29 28 27 26 25 (48 47 46 45 44 43 42 41)	24 23 22 21 20 19 18 17 (31 32 33 34 35 36 37 38)

PART 1: CHAPTER WORD JUMBLES

Note: Answers can be obtained from your instructor and their Evolve Resources

Chapter 1: Face and Neck Regions

1. *Lower jaw* LEDIBMAN ☐☐☐☐☐☐☐☐
2. *Ramus part* ONORIDCO ☐☐☐☐☐☐☐☐
3. *Kisser corner* SUREMISCOM ☐☐☐☐☐☐☐☐☐☐
4. *Muscle mania* TERSEMAS ☐☐☐☐☐☐☐☐
5. *In thyroid* DOIRTHYARAP ☐☐☐☐☐☐☐☐☐☐☐
6. *Cheeky gland* TIDROPA ☐☐☐☐☐☐☐
7. *Upper lip thick* UERBCLET ☐☐☐☐☐☐☐☐
8. *Upper lip dip* TURIMLPH ☐☐☐☐☐☐☐☐
9. *Head joint* MANBTOROPDIULAREM ☐☐☐☐☐☐☐☐☐☐☐☐☐☐☐☐☐
10. *Lipstick home* LIONMIREV ☐☐☐☐☐☐☐☐☐

Chapter 2: Oral Cavity and Pharynx

1. *Misplaced oil* ODRCYEF ☐☐☐☐☐☐☐
2. *Dog teeth* NESNICA ☐☐☐☐☐☐☐
3. *Grinding fun* CASTIMIOATN ☐☐☐☐☐☐☐☐☐☐☐
4. *Arch bumps* SESXTOESO ☐☐☐☐☐☐☐☐☐
5. *Tooth padding* VAINGGI ☐☐☐☐☐☐☐
6. *Entrance walls* UFALAIC ☐☐☐☐☐☐☐
7. *Tongue specials* LALAPPIE ☐☐☐☐☐☐☐☐
8. *Tongue line-up* VALARICTMUCE ☐☐☐☐☐☐☐☐☐☐☐☐
9. *Bony arches* EORVALAL ☐☐☐☐☐☐☐☐
10. *Mushroom-shape specials* GORMFUNIF ☐☐☐☐☐☐☐☐☐

Chapter 3: Prenatal Development

1. *Cavity fluid* TICNAIMO ☐☐☐☐☐☐☐☐
2. *Outer skin layer* MEERCODT ☐☐☐☐☐☐☐☐
3. *First divisions* GEAVECLA ☐☐☐☐☐☐☐☐
4. *Genetic map* YOKAPRETY ☐☐☐☐☐☐☐☐☐
5. *Future embryo* TOYSCBALST ☐☐☐☐☐☐☐☐☐☐
6. *Union result* GOTEYZ ☐☐☐☐☐☐
7. *From ectoderm* NETUCREDMOORE ☐☐☐☐☐☐☐☐☐☐☐☐☐
8. *Embryonic tissue* CESHEMENYM ☐☐☐☐☐☐☐☐☐☐
9. *First draft* RORPUDMIMI ☐☐☐☐☐☐☐☐☐☐
10. *Toxic types* EGRAOENTTS ☐☐☐☐☐☐☐☐☐☐

Chapter 4: Face and Neck Development

1. *Nose bump* RACTIEGAL ☐☐☐☐☐☐☐☐☐
2. *Gill time* CHIALRANB ☐☐☐☐☐☐☐☐☐
3. *Disappearance act* KEECLM ☐☐☐☐☐☐
4. *Neck bone* DIHOY ☐☐☐☐☐
5. *Sense button* DLAPSECO ☐☐☐☐☐☐☐☐
6. *Outer doughnut part* RATELLA ☐☐☐☐☐☐☐
7. *Opening gives communication* NEEMBARM ☐☐☐☐☐☐☐☐
8. *Four evaginations* CPHOSUE ☐☐☐☐☐☐☐
9. *Upper facial place* SOOFNTNAARL ☐☐☐☐☐☐☐☐☐☐☐
10. *Primitive oral landmark* MTOODEMUS ☐☐☐☐☐☐☐☐☐

Chapter 5: Orofacial Development

1. *Tight tongue* AAGYOINSSKLOL ☐☐☐☐☐☐☐☐☐☐☐☐☐
2. *Parting palate* LETCF ☐☐☐☐☐
3. *From fourth swelling* TEIPLIGOCT ☐☐☐☐☐☐☐☐☐☐
4. *Stacked six* IESGLWLNS ☐☐☐☐☐☐☐☐☐

5. *Funny throat thing* AULVU ⬚⬚⬚⬚⬚

6. *Overgrowing base* OUPALC ⬚⬚⬚⬚⬚⬚

7. *Middle meeting* LESVHSE ⬚⬚⬚⬚⬚⬚⬚

8. *Roof parts* AALPLAT ⬚⬚⬚⬚⬚⬚⬚

9. *Initial tongue blob* RETMCUBUUL ⬚⬚⬚⬚⬚⬚⬚⬚⬚⬚

10. *In midline* AIPRM ⬚⬚⬚⬚⬚

Chapter 6: Tooth Development and Eruption

1. *Empty slot* OOAANDINT ⬚⬚⬚⬚⬚⬚⬚⬚⬚

2. *Leftover cells* ZELSMAAS ⬚⬚⬚⬚⬚⬚⬚⬚

3. *Twining trouble* NOIEGMIATN ⬚⬚⬚⬚⬚⬚⬚⬚⬚⬚

4. *Primary shedders* STOSLAODNTOC ⬚⬚⬚⬚⬚⬚⬚⬚⬚⬚⬚⬚

5. *Early bony-like form* IOMCEETND ⬚⬚⬚⬚⬚⬚⬚⬚⬚

6. *Secretory surface* SMTEO ⬚⬚⬚⬚⬚

7. *Compressed layer* MMDIUNTREEI ⬚⬚⬚⬚⬚⬚⬚⬚⬚⬚⬚

8. *Second draft* NUUCDSCEAEOS ⬚⬚⬚⬚⬚⬚⬚⬚⬚⬚⬚⬚

9. *Merry myth* YIFAR ⬚⬚⬚⬚⬚

10. *Accessory cusps* BEECLSTUR ⬚⬚⬚⬚⬚⬚⬚⬚⬚

Chapter 7: Cells

1. *Cytoplasm spaces* VAUCLEOS ⬚⬚⬚⬚⬚⬚⬚⬚

2. *Splitting up* SOMTIIS ⬚⬚⬚⬚⬚⬚⬚

3. *Junction tie* DOSMMEOSE ⬚⬚⬚⬚⬚⬚⬚⬚⬚

4. *Cell center* ULCELOUNS ⬚⬚⬚⬚⬚⬚⬚⬚⬚

5. *Moving out* OSSEYTOXIC ⬚⬚⬚⬚⬚⬚⬚⬚⬚⬚

6. *Breaking down* MESYSLOOS ⬚⬚⬚⬚⬚⬚⬚⬚⬚

7. *Chromatin condenses* ROSHAEPP ⬚⬚⬚⬚⬚⬚⬚⬚

8. *Two chromatids* TEMRONEECR ⬚⬚⬚⬚⬚⬚⬚⬚⬚⬚

9. *Rough guys* SRIMBOOES ⬚⬚⬚⬚⬚⬚⬚⬚⬚

10. *Major player* FEMSTOINNOLAT ⬚⬚⬚⬚⬚⬚⬚⬚⬚⬚⬚⬚⬚

Chapter 8: Basic Tissue

1. *Mineral identification* PAAYTHRIODXYTE ☐☐☐☐☐☐☐☐☐☐☐☐☐☐
2. *Nutrition canals* CIALNAULIC ☐☐☐☐☐☐☐☐☐
3. *Vessel wrapping* THELENDOMUI ☐☐☐☐☐☐☐☐☐☐☐
4. *Layered epithelium* EFADISTRTI ☐☐☐☐☐☐☐☐☐
5. *Hard rings* TONESSO ☐☐☐☐☐☐☐
6. *Making fibers* BIABSLFROT ☐☐☐☐☐☐☐☐☐☐
7. *Alien stuff* NIOMUMENG ☐☐☐☐☐☐☐☐☐
8. *Replacement clocking* ORVENTUR ☐☐☐☐☐☐☐☐
9. *Clot creation* TELLEPAST ☐☐☐☐☐☐☐☐☐
10. *Nerve communication* NYSASEP ☐☐☐☐☐☐☐

Chapter 9: Oral Mucosa

1. *Unique tissue* TEZEKPAIRNADAIR ☐☐☐☐☐☐☐☐☐☐☐☐☐☐☐
2. *Waterproofing tactic* RAKTENI ☐☐☐☐☐☐☐
3. *Dark spots* LUGREANS ☐☐☐☐☐☐☐☐
4. *Gum tufting* TIGPIPSLN ☐☐☐☐☐☐☐☐☐
5. *Blood group* ACALPRILY ☐☐☐☐☐☐☐☐☐
6. *Down deeper* BOSSAMUUC ☐☐☐☐☐☐☐☐☐
7. *Italy map* PHIRGAEOCG ☐☐☐☐☐☐☐☐☐☐
8. *Membrane with bony down under* SMUMEPOCEIROTU ☐☐☐☐☐☐☐☐☐☐☐☐☐☐
9. *Tongue field* ZISPAEECLID ☐☐☐☐☐☐☐☐☐☐☐
10. *Dried up* KEPICRL ☐☐☐☐☐☐☐

Chapter 10: Gingival and Dentogingival Junctional Tissue

1. *Between layers* NALAMI ☐☐☐☐☐☐
2. *Facing tooth* LAVDENINGTOGI ☐☐☐☐☐☐☐☐☐☐☐☐☐
3. *Always young* JOUCTIANNL ☐☐☐☐☐☐☐☐☐☐

4. *Periodontal playground* LUULSCRA ☐☐☐☐☐☐☐☐

5. *Future fluid measurement* VUCRRIECLA ☐☐☐☐☐☐☐☐☐☐

6. *Growing gums* HYSAPARLEPI ☐☐☐☐☐☐☐☐☐☐☐

7. *Longer teeth* CORSEESIN ☐☐☐☐☐☐☐☐☐

8. *Sore gums* TIINVSGIGI ☐☐☐☐☐☐☐☐☐☐

9. *Deeper disease* KEOPCT ☐☐☐☐☐☐

10. *Continued infection* DIREPOONTIITS ☐☐☐☐☐☐☐☐☐☐☐☐☐

Chapter 11: Head and Neck Structures

1. *Group secretion* SANCIU ☐☐☐☐☐☐

2. *Gland masses* ELFSOLILC ☐☐☐☐☐☐☐☐☐

3. *Node depression* HUISL ☐☐☐☐☐

4. *Bigger grapes* PYHMDAPELONTYAH ☐☐☐☐☐☐☐☐☐☐☐☐☐☐☐

5. *Nasal projections* OCCHENA ☐☐☐☐☐☐☐

6. *Desert place* XOOERASMTI ☐☐☐☐☐☐☐☐☐☐

7. *Head spaces* RANSPALAA ☐☐☐☐☐☐☐☐☐

8. *Damp kisser* ILASAV ☐☐☐☐☐☐

9. *Making thyroxine* DOLICLO ☐☐☐☐☐☐☐

10. *Lymphoid masses* TALOLNSIR ☐☐☐☐☐☐☐☐☐

Chapter 12: Enamel

1. *Breaking crystals* FABTCANRIO ☐☐☐☐☐☐☐☐☐☐

2. *Dark brushes* FUSTT ☐☐☐☐☐

3. *Rubbed out* BANRAISO ☐☐☐☐☐☐☐☐

4. *Faulty enamel* PDSSYILAA ☐☐☐☐☐☐☐☐☐

5. *Short tubules* NIESDSPL ☐☐☐☐☐☐☐☐

6. *Named layers* TRIESZU ☐☐☐☐☐☐☐

7. *Hard rock bands* AICTMBRINIO ☐☐☐☐☐☐☐☐☐☐☐

8. *Worn jewel* NOTATRITI ☐☐☐☐☐☐☐☐☐

9. *Between enamel units* DORNITER ☐☐☐☐☐☐☐☐

10. *Outer grooviness* KYMPERATIA ☐☐☐☐☐☐☐☐☐☐

Chapter 13: Dentin and Pulp

1. *Whole hole* MONFRAE ☐☐☐☐☐☐☐
2. *Disturbed appositional growth* TURCONO ☐☐☐☐☐☐☐
3. *Around middle* CUCPIRAUMPLL ☐☐☐☐☐☐☐☐☐☐☐
4. *First covering* NETMAL ☐☐☐☐☐☐
5. *Around tubes* BUTLERAPIUR ☐☐☐☐☐☐☐☐☐☐
6. *Tubule type* TNADELIN ☐☐☐☐☐☐☐☐
7. *Lateral complications* RAOSCECSY ☐☐☐☐☐☐☐☐☐
8. *Avoid ice* VEISHYPIERSNITTY ☐☐☐☐☐☐☐☐☐☐☐☐☐☐☐☐
9. *Named layers* BERNE ☐☐☐☐☐
10. *Inner pain* TULSPIPI ☐☐☐☐☐☐☐☐

Chapter 14: Periodontium: Cementum, Alveolar Process, and Periodontal Ligament

1. *Trouble scaling* PURSS ☐☐☐☐☐
2. *No cells* RACELALUL ☐☐☐☐☐☐☐☐☐
3. *Two kinds* NELMSECTICE ☐☐☐☐☐☐☐☐☐☐☐
4. *Dental nightmare* EUSUDENTOL ☐☐☐☐☐☐☐☐☐☐
5. *Bulk fibers* QUOIBLE ☐☐☐☐☐☐☐
6. *Extra extra* ISHTYMERCEPENSO ☐☐☐☐☐☐☐☐☐☐☐☐☐☐☐
7. *Probing junction* MEECLEMENTONA ☐☐☐☐☐☐☐☐☐☐☐☐☐
8. *Between roots* RACDILTERIUARN ☐☐☐☐☐☐☐☐☐☐☐☐☐☐
9. *Supporting team* TERIMOODPINU ☐☐☐☐☐☐☐☐☐☐☐☐
10. *Ninety degrees* YESHARP ☐☐☐☐☐☐☐

Chapter 15: Overview of Dentitions

1. *Meeting place* TACONCT ☐☐☐☐☐☐☐
2. *Floss heaven* INOXTMERPRIAL ☐☐☐☐☐☐☐☐☐☐☐☐☐
3. *Bite me* SOONCLUIC ☐☐☐☐☐☐☐☐☐
4. *Ortho charting* LEPARM ☐☐☐☐☐☐

5. *Four squares* DANQTUARNS ⬜⬜⬜⬜⬜⬜⬜⬜⬜⬜

6. *Linear elevations* GRISED ⬜⬜⬜⬜⬜⬜

7. *Root caves* VITANESCOCI ⬜⬜⬜⬜⬜⬜⬜⬜⬜⬜⬜

8. *Six slices* XSASENTT ⬜⬜⬜⬜⬜⬜⬜⬜

9. *More specific* HIRSTD ⬜⬜⬜⬜⬜⬜

10. *Talking points* AUSLNIVER ⬜⬜⬜⬜⬜⬜⬜⬜⬜

Chapter 16: Permanent Anterior Teeth

1. *Traumatic injury* NALVUISO ⬜⬜⬜⬜⬜⬜⬜⬜

2. *Backside booty* CUIMGLUN ⬜⬜⬜⬜⬜⬜⬜⬜

3. *Older dog tooth term* DUCSPI ⬜⬜⬜⬜⬜⬜

4. *Cute space* STIEAMAD ⬜⬜⬜⬜⬜⬜⬜⬜

5. *Odd incisor* CHONTUSHIN ⬜⬜⬜⬜⬜⬜⬜⬜⬜⬜

6. *Getting depressed* SOAFSE ⬜⬜⬜⬜⬜⬜

7. *Canine retained* PIAMDCET ⬜⬜⬜⬜⬜⬜⬜⬜

8. *New ridge* SIACLIN ⬜⬜⬜⬜⬜⬜⬜

9. *Even cuter* LOESMNAM ⬜⬜⬜⬜⬜⬜⬜⬜

10. *Extra something* EOSEDIMNS ⬜⬜⬜⬜⬜⬜⬜⬜⬜

Chapter 17: Permanent Posterior Teeth

1. *Older molar friend term* SPUDICIB ⬜⬜⬜⬜⬜⬜⬜⬜

2. *Maxillary special* QOEUBIL ⬜⬜⬜⬜⬜⬜⬜

3. *Cute cusp* CLERIABAL ⬜⬜⬜⬜⬜⬜⬜⬜⬜

4. *Angular distortion* LEDIARTOCAIN ⬜⬜⬜⬜⬜⬜⬜⬜⬜⬜⬜⬜

5. *Elongated depression* TULFGINT ⬜⬜⬜⬜⬜⬜⬜⬜

6. *Hidden areas* SHERCOTC ⬜⬜⬜⬜⬜⬜⬜⬜

7. *Odd molar* BUMLYRER ⬜⬜⬜⬜⬜⬜⬜⬜

8. *Outside deep groove* UFINSO ⬜⬜⬜⬜⬜⬜

9. *Between roots* AURCFINOT ⬜⬜⬜⬜⬜⬜⬜⬜⬜

10. *Three roots* TERICFRATUD ⬜⬜⬜⬜⬜⬜⬜⬜⬜⬜⬜

Chapter 18: Primary Dentition

1. *Baby spaces* MIPERAT ☐☐☐☐☐☐☐
2. *Prominent ridge* RIAVCECL ☐☐☐☐☐☐☐☐
3. *Large chamber* LUPP ☐☐☐☐
4. *Risky restorative moment* NORSH ☐☐☐☐☐
5. *Early childhood* SECAIR ☐☐☐☐☐☐
6. *Stained teeth* NAMTHYS ☐☐☐☐☐☐☐
7. *Good start teeth* MRIYPAR ☐☐☐☐☐☐☐
8. *Kid grinding* XIRSBUM ☐☐☐☐☐☐☐
9. *Worn tops* OARNTTITI ☐☐☐☐☐☐☐☐☐
10. *Whiter baby smile* EELANM ☐☐☐☐☐☐

Chapter 19: Temporomandibular Joint

1. *Raising mandible* VEAOINLET ☐☐☐☐☐☐☐☐☐
2. *Inferior depression* CAARITLUR ☐☐☐☐☐☐☐☐☐
3. *Joint fluid* YNOILVSA ☐☐☐☐☐☐☐☐
4. *Side movement* TELLARA ☐☐☐☐☐☐☐
5. *Working muscles* MOICTASAITN ☐☐☐☐☐☐☐☐☐☐☐
6. *Sharper ridge* GLOPOSTEDIN ☐☐☐☐☐☐☐☐☐☐☐
7. *Partial dislocation* BUIULXATSON ☐☐☐☐☐☐☐☐☐☐☐
8. *Joint change* SRIDDORE ☐☐☐☐☐☐☐☐
9. *Joint cover* LEAPSCU ☐☐☐☐☐☐☐
10. *Jaw backward* TROINRACTE ☐☐☐☐☐☐☐☐☐☐

Chapter 20: Occlusion

1. *Noisy occlusion* MRUIBXS ☐☐☐☐☐☐☐
2. *Mandible facial* TROSBSICE ☐☐☐☐☐☐☐☐☐
3. *Lateral curve* NOLSIW ☐☐☐☐☐☐
4. *Resting mandible* RLEANECAC ☐☐☐☐☐☐☐☐☐
5. *Space for kids* WEEYLA ☐☐☐☐☐☐
6. *Major disharmony* MRATAU ☐☐☐☐☐☐
7. *Habitually centric* OINCUCLSO ☐☐☐☐☐☐☐☐☐
8. *More women* ROIVEEBT ☐☐☐☐☐☐☐☐
9. *Horizontal overhang* JOEVETR ☐☐☐☐☐☐☐
10. *Occlusal classification* GALNE ☐☐☐☐☐

PART 2: UNIT CROSSWORD PUZZLES

Note: Answers can be obtained from your Instructor and their Evolve Resources

UNIT I: OROFACIAL STRUCTURES

Crossword, Puzzle 1

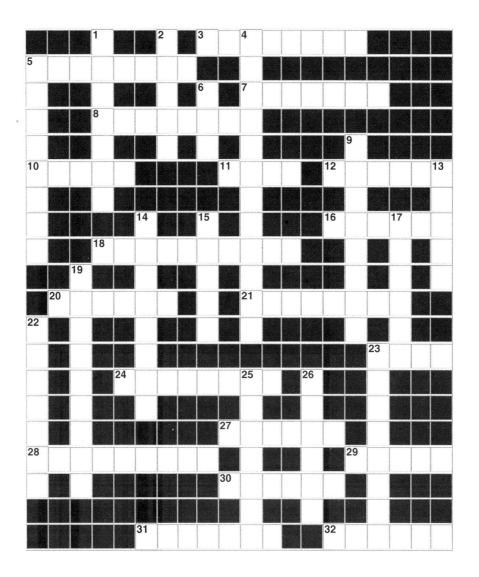

Across:

3 Vertical groove noted on midline of upper lip

5 Bony process at anterior border of mandibular ramus

7 Small yellowish oral mucosal elevations from misplaced sebaceous glands

8 Part of maxilla or mandible that supports teeth

10 Nostrils of nose

11 External main feature of nasal region so do not blow it!

12 Structures or facial surfaces of a tooth closest to inner cheek

16 Alveolar process between two neighboring teeth, also called *interdental*

18 Part of the face that contains the lips and oral cavity

20 Hard inner crown layer of tooth overlying pulp

21 Socket of tooth

23 White ridge of raised keratinized epithelial tissue on buccal mucosa

24 Lower jaw

27 Hard outer crown layer of tooth

28 Variation in bone growth on facial surface of maxillary alveolar process

29 Skull socket that contains eyeball and supporting structures

30 Space facing the sulcular epithelium

31 Bony projection off posterior and superior border of mandibular ramus

32 Voice box in the midline of neck that is composed of cartilages

Down:

1 Opening from the pulp at the apex of the tooth

2 Keratinization on inner cheek where the teeth occlude

4 Facial region located both inferior to orbital region and lateral to nasal region

5 Outermost layer of the root of a tooth

6 Winglike cartilaginous structure laterally around each nares

9 Midline thickening of the upper lip

13 Tissue fluid that drains from surrounding region into lymphatic vessels

14 Small elevated structures of specialized mucosa on the tongue

15 Depression located where sulcus terminalis points backward toward pharynx

17 Nonencapsulated mass of lymphoid tissue

19 Darker appearance or zone of the lips compared with surrounding skin

22 Anteriors that are also the third teeth from the midline in each quadrant

23 Teeth type that includes incisors and canines located at the front of oral cavity

25 Describes structures or tooth surfaces closest to the tongue

26 Midline tissue fold between ventral surface of the tongue and floor of the mouth

UNIT II: DENTAL EMBRYOLOGY

Crossword, Puzzle 1

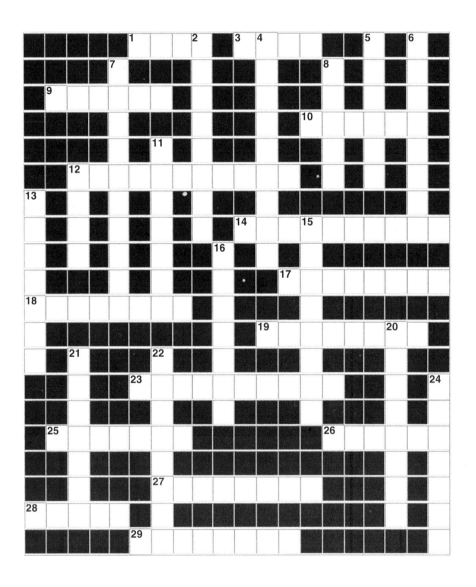

Across:

1 Circular plate of bilayered cells developed from the blastocyst

3 Depressions in the center of each nasal placode that evolve into the nasal cavities

9 Elimination of this structure between two adjacent swellings during surface fusion

10 Type of tube formed when neural folds meet and fuse superior to the neural groove

12 Cells that differentiate from preameloblasts forming enamel during amelogenesis

14 Overall form of a structure that can undergo change during development

17 Embryonic layer located between ectoderm and endoderm

18 Superior layer in the bilaminar embryonic disc

19 Areas of ectoderm found located at developing special sense organs on embryo

23 Embryonic disc that includes the ectoderm, mesoderm, and endoderm

25 Intermaxillary growth from paired medial nasal processes on internal stomodeum

26 Tail end of a structure such as with the trilaminar embryonic disc

27 Each half of it mirrors the other half of the embryo due to primitive streak development

28 Structure of the fetal period of prenatal development derived from enlarged embryo

29 Process during prenatal development when mitosis converts a zygote to a blastocyst

Down:

2 Head end of a structure such as with the trilaminar embryonic disc

4 Action of one cell group on another leading to establishment of developmental pathway

5 Structure derived from the implanted blastocyst

6 Posterior one develops from fourth branchial arches marking future epiglottis

7 Developmental problems evident at birth

8 Specialized cells that develop from neuroectoderm that migrate from the neural folds

11 Paired cuboidal aggregates of cells differentiated from the mesoderm

12 Branchial apparatus part that includes these as well as grooves, membranes, and pouches

13 Cleft lip is fusion failure of the maxillary one with the medial nasal one on each side

15 Processes that occur from the start of pregnancy to birth

16 Membrane at the caudal end of the embryo that is the future anus

20 Trilaminar embryonic disc layer derived from the epiblast layer that lines stomodeum

21 Anterior part of future digestive tract or primitive pharynx forming oropharynx

22 Membrane that disintegrates bringing nasal and oral cavities into communication

24 Process occurring to embryo that places each embryologic tissue in proper position

UNIT II: DENTAL EMBRYOLOGY

Crossword, Puzzle 2

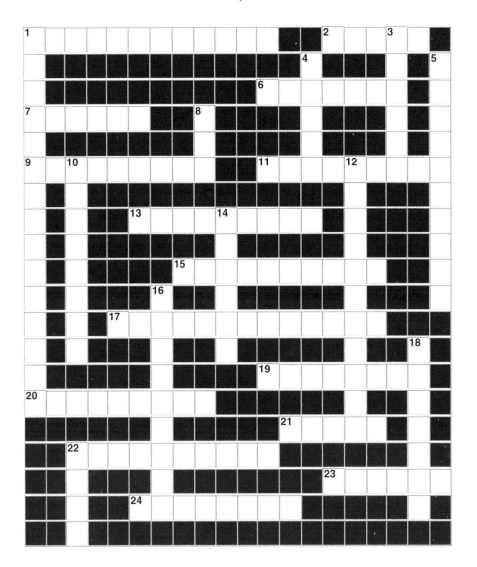

Across:

1 Canals that persist after development

2 Fusion failure of palatal shelves with the primary palate or with each other

6 Two palatal processes from the maxillary processes during prenatal development

7 Part of cervical loop that shape root or roots inducing root dentin formation

9 Cementum matrix laid down by cementoblasts

11 Circular plate of bilayered cells developed from the blastocyst

13 One cell group action that leads to developmental pathway in responding tissue

15 Layered formation of tissue such as cartilage, bone, enamel, dentin, or cementum

17 Process by which the sperm penetrates the ovum during preimplantation period

19 Photographic analysis of chromosomes

20 Primitive mouth appearing as shallow depression in embryonic surface

21 Cap or bell-shaped part of tooth germ that produces enamel

22 Prenatal structure of trophoblast cells and inner cell mass that develops into embryo

23 Substance that is partially calcified and serves as a framework for later calcification

24 Layer in the trilaminar embryonic disc derived from hypoblast layer

Down:

1 Permanent teeth type without primary predecessors that are also known as *molars*

3 Dental developmental disturbance in which adjacent tooth germs unite

4 Small spherical enamel projection near cementoenamel junction

5 Cellular removal of hard tissue such as bone, enamel, dentin, or cementum

8 Second stage of tooth development with dental lamina growth into ectomesenchyme

10 Groups of epithelial cells in periodontal ligament after disintegration of sheath

12 Abnormally small teeth

14 Posterior swellings from third and fourth branchial arches that overgrow second branchial arches

16 Dentin matrix laid down through appositional growth by the odontoblasts

18 Process of reproductive cell production that ensures correct number of chromosomes

22 Fourth stage of odontogenesis in which differentiation occurs to its furthest extent

UNIT III: DENTAL HISTOLOGY

Crossword, Puzzle 1

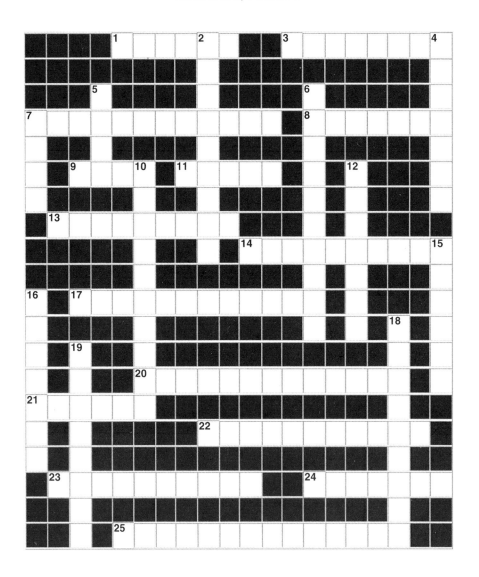

Across:

1 Group of organs functioning together

3 Closely apposed sheets of bone tissue in compact bone

7 Organelles associated with manufacture of adenosine triphosphate

8 Largest and most conspicuous organelle in the cell

9 Smallest unit of organization in the body

11 Somewhat independent part that performs a specific function or functions

13 Chief nucleoprotein in the nondividing nucleoplasm

14 White blood cell that increases in numbers during an immune response

17 Three-dimensional system of support within the cell

20 Type of intermediate filament with major role in intercellular junctions

21 Structure formed by cell groups with similar characteristics of shape and function

22 Immature connective tissue formed during initial repair

23 Filamentous daughter chromosomes joined at a centromere during cell division

24 Specialized connective tissue composed of fat, little matrix, and adipocytes

25 Along with calcium, main inorganic crystal in enamel, bone, dentin, and cementum

Down:

2 Superficial layers of skin

4 Type of protein fiber in connective tissue composed of microfilaments

5 Rigid connective tissue

6 Metabolically inert substances or transient structures within the cell

7 White blood cell similar to basophil that is also involved in allergic responses

10 Second most common white blood cell in the blood

12 Part of cell division resulting in two daughter cells identical to the parent cell

15 Small space that surrounds a chondrocyte or an osteocyte

16 Intermediate protein filament that consists of an opaque waterproof substance

18 Intercellular junction found between cells

19 White blood cell that contains granules of histamine and heparin

UNIT III: DENTAL HISTOLOGY

Crossword, Puzzle 2

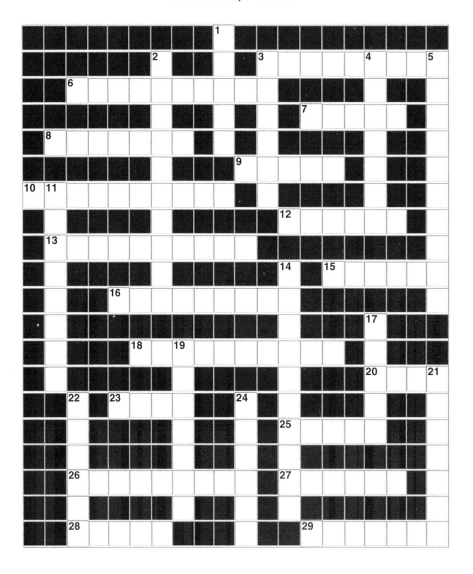

Across:

3 Tissue deep to oral mucosa composed of loose connective tissue

6 Joined matrix pieces forming lattice in cancellous bone

7 Tissue fluid that drains from the surrounding region into lymphatic vessels

8 Initially formed bone matrix

9 Central opening where saliva is deposited after production by secretory cells

10 Mature osteoblasts entrapped in bone matrix

12 Respiratory mucosal cells that produce mucus to keep mucosa moist

13 Network of vessels that collect and transport lymph linking the lymph nodes

15 Hard tooth tissue loss from demineralization by cariogenic bacteria

16 Blood cell fragments that function in clotting mechanism

18 Dense connective tissue layer on outer part of bone

20 Extension or "peg" of the epithelium into connective tissue in microscopic section

23 Passageway that allows glandular secretion to be emptied directly into location of use

25 Large inner part of certain glands

26 Dense connective tissue in both dermis and lamina propria

27 Secretion from salivary glands that lubricates and cleanses oral cavity

28 Bundle of neural processes outside the central nervous system

29 Localized macules of pigmentation

Down:

1 Depression on one side of the lymph node

2 Grooves associated with lines of Retzius in enamel

3 Connective tissue that divides inner part of certain glands

4 Connective tissue that surrounds outer part of entire gland or lesion

5 Cells that differentiate from preameloblasts forming enamel during amelogenesis

11 Epithelium that stands away from the tooth creating a gingival sulcus

14 Cells that function in resorption of bone

17 Nostril of nose

19 Incremental lines located in histologic preparations of mature enamel

21 Hard tooth tissue loss through chemical means not involving bacteria

22 Functional cellular component of the nervous system

24 Extracellular substance that serves as framework for later calcification

UNIT III: DENTAL HISTOLOGY

Crossword, Puzzle 3

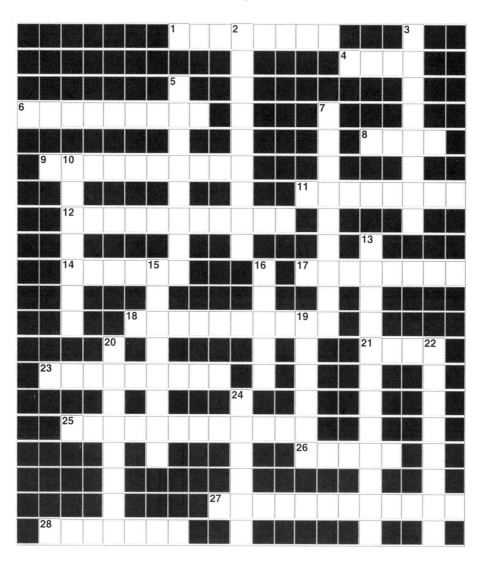

Across:

1   Inflammation of pulp

4   Soft innermost connective tissue in both the crown and root

6   Hard tooth tissue loss by mastication or parafunctional habits

8   Crystalline structural units of enamel that gives teeth the bright white

9   Layered formation of firm or hard tissue such as enamel, dentin, or cementum

11   Surrounds the teeth for support and attaches the teeth to the alveoli

12   Incremental lines or bands of von Ebner in mature dentin

14   Opening or foramen from the pulp at apex

17   Socket of tooth

18   Cancellous bone located between alveolar bone proper and plates of cortical bone

21   Imbrication lines in dentin demonstrating disturbance in body metabolism

23   Extra openings usually located on the lateral parts of the roots

25   Appositional growth of enamel matrix by ameloblasts

26   Microscopic dark brushes in enamel with bases near the dentinoenamel junction

27   Layer of dentin around the outer pulpal wall

28   Part of the tooth that contains the mass of pulp

Down:

2   Dentin matrix laid down by appositional growth by the odontoblasts

3   Microscopic enamel feature of short dentinal tubules near the dentinoenamel junction

5   Plates of compact bone on the facial and lingual surfaces of the alveolar process

7   Part of the pulp located in the root area of the tooth

10   Dentin formed in a tooth before the completion of the apical foramen

13   Supporting hard or soft dental tissue for the tooth

15   Hard tooth tissue loss by friction from toothbrushing and/or toothpaste

16   Found within dentinal tubule in dentin

19   Smooth microscopic lines in cartilage, bone, or cementum due to appositional growth

20   Outermost layer of root of a tooth

22   Accentuated incremental line of Retzius or contour line of Owen from birth process

24   Hard inner layer of the crown of a tooth overlying pulp

UNIT IV: DENTAL ANATOMY

Crossword, Puzzle 1

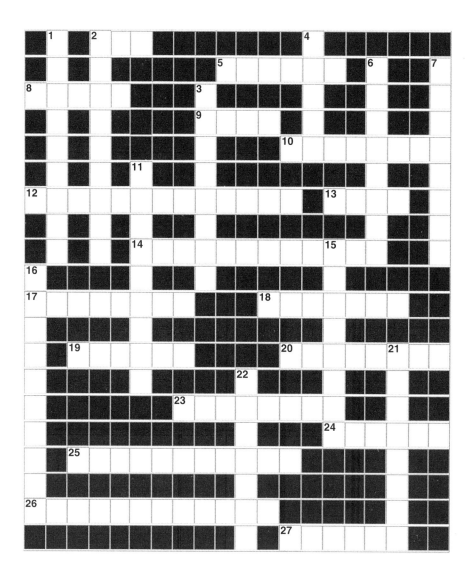

Across:

2 Small lateral incisor or third molar crown due to partial microdontia

5 Palmer Notation _____

8 Mythological night time creature that takes shed primary teeth leaving cold hard cash

9 Type of angle formed by lines created at junction of two crown surfaces

10 Rounded enamel extensions on anterior incisal ridge as noted from labial or lingual

12 Tooth designation system using a two-digit code

13 Imaginary line representing a long line of a tooth that bisects the cervical line

14 Crown or root(s) that show angular distortion

17 Rounded raised borders on mesial and distal parts of lingual surface of anteriors

18 Older dental term for canines with much thanks to our tail-wagging friends

19 Surface of a tooth closest to midline

20 Masticatory surface of posteriors

23 Vertically oriented and labially placed bony ridges of the alveolar process in both jaws

24 Surface of tooth farthest away from midline

25 Indentations on surface of the root or roots

26 Secondary groove on lingual surface of anteriors and occlusal table on posteriors

27 Division of a crown surface or root into three parts

Down:

1 Division of each dental arch into two parts with four for entire dentition

2 Second dentition noted in oral cavity also known as *adult teeth*

3 Part of root visible to the clinician

4 Depression on lingual surface of anteriors or occlusal table of posteriors

6 Complete displacement of the tooth from the socket due to extensive trauma

7 Open contact existing between maxillary central incisors

11 Absence of a single tooth or multiple teeth due to lack of initiation

15 Unerupted or partially erupted tooth positioned against an oral structure

16 Spaces formed from the curvatures where two teeth in the same arch contact

21 Division of each dental arch into three parts based on midline

22 Linear elevation or ridge on masticatory surface of newly erupted incisors

UNIT IV: DENTAL ANATOMY

Crossword, Puzzle 2

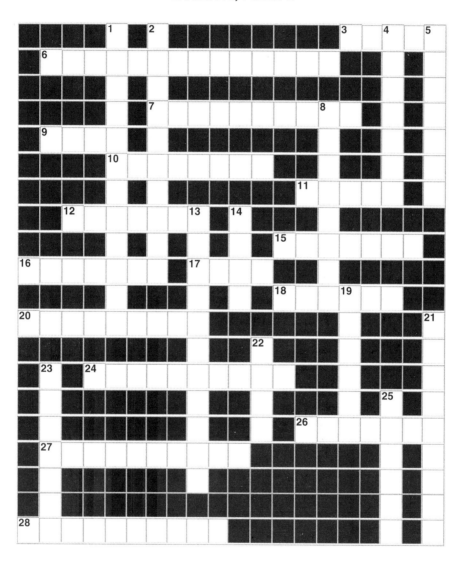

Across:

3 Situation in which entire posterior quadrant functions during lateral occlusion

6 Movements of the mandible that are not within the usual patterns

7 Moving lower jaw forward

9 Temporomandibular joint part between temporal bone and mandibular condyle

10 Ridge running mesiodistally in the cervical one third of the buccal crown surface

11 Natural movement of all of the teeth over time toward the midline of the oral cavity

12 Parafunctional habit of grinding teeth that sounds like a jet taking off

15 First dentition also known as *deciduous dentition*

16 Side to which the mandible has been moved during lateral occlusion

17 Terminal plane with primary mandibular second molar mesial to the maxillary molar

18 Space when primary molars are shed, making room for permanent premolars

20 Contralateral side of the arch from working side during lateral occlusion

24 Prominent mandible with normal or even retrusive maxilla and concave profile

26 End point of closure of the mandible with it in its most retruded position

27 Lowering of lower jaw

28 Moving lower jaw backward

Down:

1 Failure to have overall ideal form of the dentition while in centric occlusion

2 Cusps that function during centric occlusion

4 Maxillary dental arch facially overhangs the mandibular arch

5 Specific spaces between certain primary teeth

8 Situation in which the maxillary incisors overlap the mandibular incisors

13 Facial profile in centric occlusion with slightly protruded jaws

14 Plane where maxillary arch is convex occlusally and mandibular arch concave

19 Concave curve that results when a frontal section is taken through each molar set

21 Parafunctional habit with teeth held in centric occlusion for long periods

22 Situation in which the canine is the only tooth in function during lateral occlusion

23 Bony projection off posterior and superior borders of the mandibular ramus

25 What can occur to the periodontium and that can result from occlusal disharmony

PART 3: UNIT WORD SEARCH PUZZLES

UNIT I: OROFACIAL STRUCTURES

Words to Find

ALA
ANGLE
APEX
ARTICULATING
BUCCAL
COMMISSURE
CONDYLE
CORONOID
FRONTAL
HYOID

INFRAORBITAL
LABIOMENTAL
LARYNX
LYMPH
MANDIBLE
MASSETER
MENTAL
NARIS
NASAL
NOSE

ORBIT
PARATHYROID
PAROTID
PHILTRUM
PROPORTIONS
RAMUS
ROOT
STERNOCLEIDOMASTOID
SUBLINGUAL
SUBMANDIBULAR

SUBMENTAL
SULCUS
SYMPHYSIS
TEMPOROMANDIBULAR
THYROID
TUBERCLE
VERMILION
ZYGOMATIC

Word Search, Puzzle 1

L	A	R	Y	N	X	S	K	P	R	O	P	O	R	T	I	O	N	S	I
S	R	D	O	G	Z	H	L	A	T	N	O	R	F	T	O	O	R	D	R
I	Y	A	I	R	E	L	C	R	E	B	U	T	S	Y	L	W	I	A	Y
S	S	E	L	O	D	I	O	R	Y	H	T	A	R	A	P	O	L	L	D
Y	S	L	A	U	Y	H	N	O	S	E	H	Q	L	O	T	U	A	I	E
H	I	Y	T	G	B	H	P	C	U	S	P	A	A	S	B	T	O	R	S
P	R	D	N	E	J	I	I	M	U	Y	I	L	A	I	I	R	U	U	B
M	A	N	E	N	W	T	D	B	Y	B	A	M	D	B	Y	S	C	L	M
Y	N	O	M	B	A	J	L	N	A	L	O	N	R	H	S	L	A	Q	A
S	H	C	B	M	A	I	E	L	A	D	A	O	T	I	U	B	V	L	S
C	J	U	O	N	N	F	O	L	I	M	A	L	M	S	I	G	A	R	S
C	I	G	G	G	K	S	M	E	B	R	O	M	N	O	X	T	B	V	E
T	Y	L	U	E	A	T	L	U	F	I	O	R	M	B	N	E	X	B	T
Z	E	A	Z	N	N	C	S	N	L	C	D	E	O	E	U	P	P	J	E
L	L	V	F	K	O	U	I	U	A	A	N	N	M	P	A	C	X	A	R
M	D	I	O	N	O	R	O	C	M	T	S	B	A	R	M	Y	C	Y	R
A	M	U	R	T	L	I	H	P	A	A	U	A	O	M	I	E	M	A	L
P	I	E	A	X	Q	M	E	L	I	S	R	T	N	J	A	N	T	U	L
E	T	C	Z	E	R	A	H	A	R	T	I	C	U	L	A	T	I	N	G
S	N	O	I	L	I	M	R	E	V	D	T	I	B	R	O	G	P	Z	V

UNIT I: OROFACIAL STRUCTURES

Words to Find

ALVEOLAR
ALVEOLUS
ANTERIOR
CARUNCLE
CECUM
DORSAL
EXOSTOSES
FACIAL
FAUCES
FAUCIAL
FILIFORM
FIMBRIATA

FOLIATE
FORDYCE
FORNIX
FUNGIFORM
GINGIVA
INCISORS
LABIAL
LINGUAL
MASTICATION
MELANIN
MOLARS
MUCOBUCCAL

MUCOGINGIVAL
MUCOSA
NASOPHARYNX
OROPHARYNX
PAROTID
PERIODONTAL
PERMANENT
POSTERIOR
PREMOLARS
PRIMARY
PTERYGOMANDIBULAR
PULP

RAPHE
RETROMOLAR
SUBMANDIBULAR
TASTE
TERMINALIS
TONSIL
TORUS
TUBEROSITY
UVULA
VENTRAL
VESTIBULES

Word Search, Puzzle 2

```
T  S  R  O  S  I  C  N  I  F  P  R  I  M  A  R  Y  F  V  T
S  L  D  E  G  N  L  M  I  L  V  S  A  Q  R  R  R  O  E  O
R  H  A  G  L  A  O  M  R  E  A  S  U  O  W  A  A  L  N  N
A  N  O  V  I  C  B  I  S  O  O  U  I  L  L  L  P  I  T  S
L  Y  U  B  I  R  N  T  T  C  F  R  G  U  O  O  H  A  R  I
O  Y  A  L  I  G  I  U  U  A  E  I  B  N  U  E  E  T  A  L
M  L  T  A  A  B  N  M  R  T  C  I  L  X  I  V  V  E  L  S
E  X  T  I  U  C  L  I  N  A  D  I  W  I  S  L  U  L  I  O
R  A  N  L  S  A  C  A  G  N  C  N  T  U  F  A  J  L  A  L
P  T  E  Y  I  O  D  U  A  O  A  E  B  S  A  T  A  S  A  R
Z  S  N  C  R  O  R  M  B  S  C  M  C  W  A  N  X  T  A  M
F  R  U  E  R  A  O  E  O  O  A  U  E  U  I  M  N  L  R  Y
P  A  O  S  N  G  H  P  B  N  C  X  M  M  M  O  O  O  F  R
F  G  A  I  Y  A  H  P  D  U  O  U  R  U  D  M  F  O  P  M
F  L  I  R  R  A  M  I  O  S  T  E  M  O  O  I  R  A  F  E
W  A  E  N  R  E  B  R  T  R  T  S  I  R  G  D  R  O  A  L
F  T  U  Y  G  U  T  O  E  A  O  R  T  N  Y  O  R  P  C  A
P  A  N  C  L  I  S  S  S  P  E  E  U  C  T  N  U  E  I  N
O  X  T  A  E  E  V  T  O  P  R  F  E  I  I  L  N  F  A  I
T  O  R  U  S  S  E  A  T  P  H  S  D  X  P  I  J  H  L  N
```

UNIT II: DENTAL EMBRYOLOGY

Words to Find

AMNIOCENTESIS
BILAMINAR
BLASTOCYST
CAUDAL
CEPHALIC
CLEAVAGE
CLOACAL
CONGENITAL
DISC

ECTODERM
EMBRYO
ENDODERM
EPIBLAST
FERTILIZATION
FETUS
FOLDING
FUSION
HYPOBLAST

INDUCTION
KARYOTYPE
MATURATION
MEIOSIS
MESODERM
MITOSIS
MORPHOLOGY
NEUROECTODERM
PRENATAL

PRIMORDIUM
SOMITES
SYMMETRY
TERATOGENS
TRILAMINAR
ZYGOTE

Word Search, Puzzle 1

```
Q F E V U D C L L S F D C L E A V A G E
A B P T X S F L M E S O D E R M S M L S
Q E I R S Y M M E T R Y B I H N R A I N
C C B I B L A S T O C Y S T E E T S O S
L T L L M I T O S I S G R G D I E I U W
O O A A W R C L V S J S O O N T T T E P
A D S M Y J A N I A E T T E N C E T R H
C E T I W D G S G T A C G E U F F D P Z
A R M N U B O D I R E N C D E P E Q R C
L M E A C I L M E O O O N C H I R J E R
M G C R E U O T R C I I P M Y D T K N O
J A B M F S Y U C N H K R O P S I U A E
F C T I X O E W M U U A I R O A L E T M
U E M U L N L A J H R R M P B B I N A B
S P D R R A Z D O Q I Y O H L X Z D L R
I H J H A A M Y I U Y O R O A S A O U Y
O A D G L Z T I G N U T D L S F T D H O
N L J I R D L I N O G Y I O T F I E Z T
K I U J S S V F O A T P U G C L O R Q B
B C Q T O C K O H N R E M Y L K N M X V
```

UNIT II: DENTAL EMBRYOLOGY

Words to Find

APPOSITION
BELL
BUD
CEMENTOBLASTS
CEMENTOCYTES
CEMENTOID
DILACERATION
ECTODERM

ECTOMESENCHYME
FUSION
GEMINATION
INDUCTION
INITIATION
MACRODONTIA
MALASSEZ
MATRIX

MEMBRANE
MICRODONTIA
MORPHOGENESIS
NONSUCCEDANEOUS
ODONTOBLASTS
ODONTOCLASTS
ORGAN
PEARL

PREAMELOBLASTS
PREDENTIN
REPOLARIZATION
RESORPTION
SHEATH
SUCCEDANEOUS
SUPERNUMERARY

Word Search, Puzzle 2

```
W  C  X  O  O  X  X  L  C  E  M  E  N  T  O  C  Y  T  E  S
M  M  A  L  A  S  S  E  Z  E  N  N  N  N  S  N  S  S  V  X
I  B  S  F  U  S  I  O  N  I  O  O  O  I  O  T  U  K  I  E
C  R  E  S  Y  G  K  A  T  I  I  I  S  I  S  O  Y  R  O  S
R  Z  X  L  P  J  R  N  T  T  T  E  T  A  E  F  T  O  T  O
O  F  P  Q  L  B  E  A  I  A  N  A  L  N  O  A  S  S  B  L
D  C  C  L  M  D  N  S  I  E  Z  B  A  E  M  N  A  X  R  N
O  E  Z  E  E  I  O  T  G  I  O  D  V  C  H  L  W  A  A  S
N  M  M  R  M  P  I  O  R  L  E  E  N  T  B  F  E  G  O  U
T  E  P  E  P  N  H  A  E  C  Z  O  A  O  M  P  R  I  D  P
I  N  G  A  I  P  L  M  C  G  I  E  T  M  A  O  R  N  O  E
A  T  D  D  R  O  A  U  Q  T  H  N  K  E  C  C  E  D  N  R
R  O  U  O  P  E  S  J  A  S  O  O  B  S  R  E  S  U  T  N
O  B  M  E  R  N  L  R  H  D  E  H  M  E  O  M  O  C  O  U
E  L  R  P  O  Q  E  S  O  T  Y  Q  R  N  D  E  R  T  C  M
K  A  W  N  E  C  E  B  M  Q  N  D  M  C  O  N  P  I  L  E
I  S  R  C  A  E  C  T  O  D  E  R  M  H  N  T  T  O  A  R
R  T  U  L  N  E  Q  L  J  M  D  F  B  Y  T  O  I  N  S  A
A  S  I  S  D  P  B  I  O  Y  P  C  U  M  I  I  O  F  T  R
C  D  J  A  S  U  W  R  V  E  E  R  T  E  A  D  N  H  S  Y
```

UNIT III: DENTAL HISTOLOGY

Words to Find

CELL
CENTROMERE
CENTROSOME
CHROMATIDS
CHROMATIN
CHROMOSOMES
CYTOPLASM
CYTOSKELETON
DESMOSOME

ENDOCYTOSIS
EXOCYTOSIS
HEMIDESMOSOME
HISTOLOGY
INCLUSIONS
INTERPHASE
KERATIN
LYSOSOMES
METAPHASE

MICROFILAMENTS
MICROTUBULES
MITOCHONDRIA
MITOSIS
NUCLEOLUS
NUCLEOPLASM
NUCLEUS
ORGAN
PHAGOCYTOSIS

PROPHASE
RIBOSOMES
SYSTEM
TELOPHASE
TISSUE
TONOFILAMENTS
VACUOLES

Word Search, Puzzle 1

```
M  I  M  E  K  W  Q  Q  P  H  A  G  O  C  Y  T  O  S  I  S
I  J  E  X  K  U  N  W  E  E  M  S  S  S  S  S  S  E  A  A
T  G  T  D  B  E  U  U  S  S  I  E  I  D  S  T  S  E  I  E
O  D  A  I  I  K  S  A  A  S  M  S  I  U  N  A  Q  R  M  S
S  M  P  K  K  S  H  L  O  O  O  T  L  E  H  S  D  O  E  M
I  M  H  L  I  P  P  T  S  T  A  O  M  P  E  N  S  L  S  J
S  J  A  T  O  O  Y  O  Y  M  E  A  O  M  O  O  O  A  E  S
M  I  S  L  T  C  M  C  O  L  L  R  O  H  R  U  L  M  T  N
I  N  E  Y  O  O  O  R  C  I  P  S  C  T  C  P  O  N  I  S
C  T  C  X  R  D  H  U  F  Y  O  O  N  A  O  S  E  T  N  V
R  E  E  H  N  C  N  O  X  M  T  E  V  E  O  M  A  O  W  E
O  R  C  E  P  H  R  G  S  I  C  O  L  M  A  R  I  L  R  C
T  P  I  C  F  C  I  E  M  N  U  C  S  L  E  S  L  E  T  H
U  H  G  B  I  N  D  S  A  U  U  E  I  K  U  L  M  N  Z  R
B  A  S  M  O  I  U  G  T  N  D  F  I  L  E  O  S  S  T  O
U  S  M  S  M  S  R  C  B  O  O  L  C  C  R  L  F  Y  O  M
L  E  R  E  W  O  O  M  L  N  L  N  R  T  H  P  E  S  A  A
E  V  H  O  O  Q  Z  M  O  E  I  O  N  M  B  N  H  T  D  T
S  D  D  Z  D  I  Q  T  E  C  U  E  G  R  T  H  J  E  O  I
L  Y  S  O  S  O  M  E  S  S  C  S  X  Y  Z  N  V  M  O  N
```

UNIT III: DENTAL HISTOLOGY

Words to Find

ADIPOSE
APPOSITIONAL
BASOPHIL
BONE
CANALICULI
CARTILAGE
CHONDROBLASTS
CHONDROCYTES

COLLAGEN
DERMIS
ELASTIC
ENDOSTEUM
ENDOTHELIUM
EOSINOPHIL
EPIDERMIS
EPITHELIUM

FIBROBLAST
GRANULATION
HAVERSIAN
HEMIDESMOSOMES
HYDROXYAPATITE
IMMUNOGEN
IMMUNOGLOBULIN
INTERSTITIAL

KERATIN
LACUNA
LAMELLAE
LYMPHOCYTE
MACROPHAGE
MAST

Word Search, Puzzle 2

```
N E S J X J V B O N E C A R T I L A G E
M A S T E P I T H E L I U M L A C U N A
U J E I J C B D L M X B D R O Z T Z I C
W I L M J H E I U L A M E L L A E L F W
I J A M O O I M M U N O G L O B U L I N
H Z S U E N Q K V M M E P I D E R M I S
I C T N A D D E R M I S D R O K X Y G H
T L I O P R C B F O F I B R O B L A S T
G D C G P O I I F A M A C R O P H A G E
G B G E O C H E M I D E S M O S O M E S
E B R N S Y Q I W E N D O T H E L I U M
O U A H I T W C H O N D R O B L A S T S
S B N A T E Q C P V A J C O L L A G E N
I A U V I S J A D I P O S E Z S V P U C
N S L E O Y G J D S D D R K E R A T I N
O O A R N Q E W U F L Y M P H O C Y T E
P P T S A W Z S I N T E R S T I T I A L
H H I I L K C U O B I E N D O S T E U M
I I O A R F H Y D R O X Y A P A T I T E
L L N N W J Q B B I C A N A L I C U L I
```

UNIT III: DENTAL HISTOLOGY

Words to Find

ENDOCHONDRAL	ODONTOCLAST	PAPILLARY	SQUAMES
INTRAMEMBRANOUS	OSSIFICATION	PERICHONDRIUM	SUBMUCOSA
MATRIX	OSTEOBLASTS	PERIOSTEUM	SYNAPSE
MONOCYTE	OSTEOCLAST	PLASMA	TONOFILAMENTS
NERVE	OSTEOCYTES	PLATELETS	TRABECULAE
NEURON	OSTEOID	RETE	
NEUTROPHIL	OSTEONS	RETICULAR	

Word Search, Puzzle 3

```
U  S  P  L  A  S  M  A  E  L  L  I  C  O  I  O  H  X  L  Z
B  U  T  F  Z  M  F  W  P  Y  R  X  F  Z  A  T  C  D  N  L
J  B  O  Y  Y  W  N  D  L  H  W  F  J  R  S  T  I  O  A  X
I  M  N  R  V  S  Y  N  A  P  S  E  F  A  H  O  I  R  S  M
V  U  O  E  F  K  F  O  T  J  I  W  L  O  E  T  D  K  U  B
P  C  F  T  L  I  B  X  E  S  H  C  T  T  A  N  U  E  A  K
L  O  I  I  Z  N  S  O  L  D  O  W  S  C  O  A  T  W  B  U
T  S  L  C  G  T  P  F  E  E  I  O  I  H  W  S  V  T  P  Z
L  A  A  U  V  R  G  W  T  E  P  F  C  H  O  O  S  F  E  G
B  C  M  L  O  A  S  S  C  I  O  S  I  E  A  E  P  R  X
L  T  E  A  S  M  O  P  V  S  D  C  R  T  L  V  O  A  I  N
E  R  N  R  T  E  N  L  S  N  K  E  Y  C  R  N  S  P  C  E
W  A  T  G  E  M  B  O  E  R  P  C  O  E  O  Z  T  I  H  U
O  B  S  S  O  B  D  R  I  D  O  T  N  Z  O  F  E  L  O  T
N  E  X  Q  B  R  R  G  X  N  N  C  W  M  S  B  O  L  N  R
E  C  K  U  L  A  P  P  O  O  M  V  K  A  T  V  C  A  D  O
U  U  B  A  A  N  K  M  D  A  V  E  C  T  E  K  Y  R  R  P
R  L  R  M  S  O  M  O  D  J  T  P  E  R  O  G  T  Y  I  H
O  A  J  E  T  U  N  K  W  E  A  J  S  I  N  K  E  W  U  I
N  E  T  S  S  S  F  K  R  I  C  U  H  X  S  B  S  X  M  L
```

UNIT III: DENTAL HISTOLOGY

Words to Find

AFFERENT	GERMINAL	LOBES	PERIODONTITIS
CAPSULE	GINGIVITIS	LOBULES	PRICKLE
COLLOID	GOBLET	LUMEN	RECESSION
DENTOGINGIVAL	GOITER	LYMPH	STIPPLING
DUCT	GRANULATION	MASTICATORY	SULCULAR
EFFERENT	HILUS	MELANIN	SULCUS
ENDOCRINE	HYPERKERATINIZED	MUCOGINGIVAL	TASTE
EXOCRINE	JUNCTIONAL	MUCOPERIOSTEUM	
FIBROBLAST	KERATIN	MUCOSA	
FOLLICLES	KERATOHYALINE	NODES	

Word Search, Puzzle 4

```
N O D E S E G V K Y Q K A O S U L C U S
A P C K O N P E H K A U R F E L E I T P
H R O H D D M Z R G E E S N F N Y S Y T
A I L H K O U U D M T R I L I E A M C D
E C L Z L C H D C I I R A L O L R U P G
T K O U I R Y E O O C N A T B B D E N H
A L I T S I P G G O P Y A O I S E I N N
P E D D T N E Y X O H E R L E N L S O T
E S W E A E R E E O B B R L M P B I Z L
R E M N S M K Z T A I L C I P G S S A N
I G A T T U E A M F T I E I O S T V O S
O I S O E D R L P S L E T T E S I I E Z
D N T G I E A V A L U S Z C N G T L W A
O G I I K C T V O N I L E L N A U E S V
N I C N E A I F X G I R C I L B Z O U V
T V A G X P N I A J A N G U O A C L Y M
I I T I V S I M O M J O N L L U P U U N
T T O V F U Z S H N C A M W M A I M Z L
I I R A D L E P B U R M E F F E R E N T
S S Y L X E D Z M G J U N C T I O N A L
```

UNIT III: DENTAL HISTOLOGY

Words to Find

ABFRACTION
ABRASION
AMELOBLAST
AMELOGENESIS
ATTRITION
CARIES
DEMILUNE

EROSION
LYMPHADENOPATHY
LYMPHATICS
MUCOCELE
MUCOSEROUS
MYOEPITHELIAL
NARIS

PARATHYROID
PERIKYMATA
RANULA
RETZIUS
SALIVA
SECRETORY
SEPTUM

SINUSITIS
THYROGLOSSAL
THYROID
THYROXINE
TONSILS
TRABECULAE
XEROSTOMIA

Word Search, Puzzle 5

```
I  B  W  S  T  H  Y  R  O  X  I  N  E  T  T  P  E  Z  P  B
S  A  B  F  R  A  C  T  I  O  N  N  K  F  S  K  Z  E  S  S
L  C  A  R  I  E  S  I  L  H  O  G  X  Z  V  I  A  U  I  A
P  A  R  A  T  H  Y  R  O  I  D  Y  E  U  Y  L  O  S  T  T
F  G  Y  L  S  I  N  U  S  I  T  I  S  H  U  R  E  A  S  N
G  D  Y  W  H  G  I  A  M  P  S  K  T  C  E  N  M  A  O  W
Y  E  D  M  U  U  R  X  L  R  N  A  E  S  E  Y  L  I  A  S
M  M  S  S  U  B  U  M  E  Y  P  B  O  G  K  B  T  D  C  D
U  I  A  E  A  J  C  Y  R  O  A  C  O  I  O  I  S  I  I  S
C  L  L  P  N  Z  W  O  N  R  U  L  R  L  R  V  T  O  U  N
O  U  I  T  I  W  T  E  T  M  E  E  E  T  D  A  R  I  O  C
C  N  V  U  U  E  D  P  E  M  P  M  T  F  H  Y  Z  I  D  L
E  E  A  M  R  A  Q  I  A  U  A  A  R  P  H  T  S  K  Q  F
L  H  T  C  H  U  R  T  Z  U  B  P  M  T  E  O  W  M  M  X
E  G  E  P  Y  G  A  H  R  F  R  Y  U  R  R  U  Q  I  G  W
P  S  M  F  Z  X  N  E  O  Y  L  W  G  E  R  G  D  A  N  T
X  Y  U  B  Z  A  U  L  E  F  X  E  R  O  S  T  O  M  I  A
L  K  N  K  S  F  L  I  C  Q  L  L  E  T  O  N  S  I  L  S
I  E  U  V  W  F  A  A  T  H  Y  R  O  G  L  O  S  S  A  L
P  H  T  B  F  V  N  L  N  A  R  I  S  B  F  W  H  S  U  Q
```

UNIT III: DENTAL HISTOLOGY

Words to Find

ACCESSORY
ALVEOLUS
APICAL
APPOSITION
ARREST
ATTRITION
CANALICULI
CEMENTICLES
CEMENTOBLASTS
CEMENTOCYTES
CEMENTOGENESIS

CEMENTOID
CEMENTUM
CHAMBER
CIRCUMPULPAL
DENTIN
DENTINOGENESIS
EDENTULOUS
FLUID
GLOBULAR
HYPERCEMENTOSIS
HYPERSENSITIVITY

IMBRICATION
INTERGLOBULAR
INTERTUBULAR
MANTLE
NEONATAL
ODONTOBLASTS
OWEN
PERIODONTIUM
PERITUBULAR
PREDENTIN
PRIMARY

PRINCIPAL
PULP
PULPITIS
RADICULAR
SECONDARY
STONES
TERTIARY
TRABECULAR
TUBULES

Word Search, Puzzle 6

```
A T T A T Q M P N T G K O I B S A D C C
R E U L C P A U E R D A W M P T T B E H
R R B V E R N L O A E P E B R O T U M A
E T U E M I T P N B N I N R I N R B E M
S I L O E N L I A E T C H I M E I H N B
T A E L N C E T T C I A Y C A S T Z T E
C R S U T I C I A U N L P A R H I C U R
E Y P S O P E S L L O I E T Y Y O E M C
M P E C I A M E I A G N R I O P N M P E
E E R I D L E V N R E T S O D E K E R M
N R I R K C N E T Z N E E N O C A N E E
T I O C S A T D E R E R N A N E P T D N
I T D U E N O E R A S G S C T M P O E T
C U O M C A G N T D I L I C O E O C N O
L B N P O L E T U I S O T E B N S Y T B
E U T U N I N U B C F B I S L T I T I L
S L I L D C E L U U L U V S A O T E N A
U A U P A U S O L L U L I O S S I S W S
I R M A R L I U A A I A T R T I O Q R T
Y Q X L Y I S S R R D R Y Y S S N E Q S
```

UNIT IV: DENTAL ANATOMY

Words to Find

ANATOMIC
AXIS
CEMENTOENAMEL
CLINICAL
CONCAVITIES
CONTACT
CONTOUR

CUSP
DECIDUOUS
DENTITION
DISTAL
EMBRASURES
INCISAL
INTERNATIONAL

INTERPROXIMAL
MASTICATORY
MESIAL
MIDLINE
OCCLUSAL
OCCLUSION
PALMER

PERMANENT
PRIMARY
PROXIMAL
QUADRANTS
SEXTANTS
THIRDS
UNIVERSAL

Word Search, Puzzle 1

```
A  I  A  J  G  I  N  T  E  R  P  R  O  X  I  M  A  L  O  Q
T  H  I  R  D  S  T  L  T  L  R  V  F  L  Y  R  V  S  B  L
P  K  L  N  B  C  F  N  T  M  X  U  A  L  U  C  T  H  E  L
N  S  O  Z  A  A  E  G  Y  D  A  I  O  O  T  N  A  M  B  L
I  F  S  T  K  N  V  W  M  C  S  S  T  C  A  C  A  X  A  J
C  S  N  Z  A  A  U  E  O  E  O  N  T  T  C  N  K  N  I  L
T  O  V  M  B  T  N  T  M  K  O  N  X  I  E  L  O  X  A  S
C  C  R  P  S  O  I  G  E  C  V  E  C  O  C  I  U  M  L  C
H  E  U  Q  K  M  V  S  J  N  S  O  T  A  T  A  I  S  Y  E
P  N  W  S  K  I  E  D  J  Q  D  N  C  A  V  X  T  Q  A  L
L  R  L  R  P  C  R  B  U  E  E  I  N  C  O  I  N  O  A  L
W  V  I  E  R  A  S  Q  K  M  M  R  S  R  L  B  T  C  R  S
Z  C  N  M  D  L  A  U  E  R  E  B  P  T  C  U  I  I  U  Y
B  J  C  V  A  H  L  C  C  T  M  P  R  V  A  N  S  O  E  R
K  M  I  F  X  R  F  K  N  P  F  C  Y  A  I  L  U  I  E  S
Q  A  S  F  U  V  Y  I  A  I  Z  S  V  L  S  D  U  M  O  I
Z  W  A  U  X  O  N  R  J  M  S  J  C  Q  I  U  L  E  E  N
O  M  L  Q  U  A  D  R  A  N  T  S  Z  C  F  A  R  K  D  T
X  W  D  E  N  T  I  T  I  O  N  D  E  K  P  Q  Z  E  D  D
O  H  M  I  D  L  I  N  E  J  H  D  T  W  N  U  Q  X  S  P
```

UNIT IV: DENTAL ANATOMY

Words to Find

ANODONTIA	CUSPIDS	FURCATION	PEG
AVULSION	DENTIGEROUS	IMPACTED	SUPERNUMERARY
BICUSPID	DIASTEMA	MAMELONS	SUPPLEMENTAL
BIFURCATED	DILACERATION	MARGINAL	TRANSVERSE
CARABELLI	EMINENCE	MESIODENS	TRIANGULAR
CENTRAL	FLUTTING	MULBERRY	TRIFURCATED
CINGULUM	FOSSA	MULTIROOTED	TUBERCLES

Word Search, Puzzle 2

```
P  K  A  C  B  B  I  F  U  R  C  A  T  E  D  E  U  F  F  M
U  O  A  I  B  T  O  S  T  Y  E  N  L  W  D  T  D  X  R  D
S  I  Z  N  N  B  I  J  U  S  W  A  U  E  D  I  O  A  E  A
F  M  C  G  K  A  D  M  R  P  T  S  T  D  P  Y  L  T  A  Q
L  P  J  U  T  G  K  E  A  N  E  O  N  S  Q  U  A  S  Y  H
U  A  K  L  L  Z  V  I  E  I  O  R  U  P  G  C  S  G  E  F
T  C  W  U  Y  S  T  M  G  R  S  C  N  N  R  O  R  M  F  V
T  T  S  M  N  N  E  L  I  L  I  K  A  U  F  O  V  F  X  E
I  E  U  A  O  L  H  T  L  B  H  I  F  D  M  F  X  A  R  I
N  D  R  D  P  W  L  Q  D  U  R  I  Z  I  Z  E  X  I  Y  Q
G  T  O  P  D  U  Y  A  E  T  R  D  X  L  Z  I  R  G  Q  N
R  N  U  R  M  F  B  T  N  T  P  C  M  A  M  S  H  A  P  P
A  S  M  M  E  U  K  U  T  D  E  A  A  C  P  E  A  I  R  S
V  C  U  A  S  R  N  B  I  I  G  R  R  E  N  M  V  C  F  Y
A  U  L  M  I  C  D  E  G  A  S  A  G  R  G  I  U  E  J  L
P  S  B  E  O  A  H  R  E  S  L  B  I  A  O  N  L  N  X  C
P  P  E  L  D  T  L  C  R  T  Z  E  N  T  D  E  S  T  D  C
X  I  R  O  E  I  C  L  O  E  X  L  A  I  P  N  I  R  D  O
I  D  R  N  N  O  B  E  U  M  K  L  L  O  S  C  O  A  D  Y
U  S  Y  S  S  N  O  S  S  A  B  I  P  N  T  E  N  L  V  X
```

UNIT IV: DENTAL ANATOMY

Words to Find

ABFRACTION
ARTICULAR
BALANCING
BRUXISM
CAPSULE
CENTRIC
CERVICAL
CLENCHING
CONDYLE
CROSSBITE
DEPRESSION

DEVIATION
DISC
DRIFT
ELEVATION
GROUP
INTEROCCLUSAL
LEEWAY
MALOCCLUSION
MESOGNATHIC
OCCLUSION
OVERBITE

OVERJET
PARAFUNCTIONAL
PREMATURE
PRIMARY
PRIMATE
PROGNATHIC
PROTRUSION
RETRACTION
RETROGNATHIC
RISE
SPEE

STEP
SUBLUXATION
SUPPORTING
SYNOVIAL
TEMPOROMANDIBULAR
TERMINAL
TRAUMA
WILSON
WORKING

Word Search, Puzzle 3

```
A U F P R I M A T E R E T R A C T I O N
R I N T E R O C C L U S A L W I L S O N
T O N T E M P O R O M A N D I B U L A R
I P G X E L E V A T I O N P R I M A R Y
C O N D Y L E M A L O C C L U S I O N J
U S P M D S U B L U X A T I O N R I S E
L P W O R K I N G B P R O G N A T H I C
A W R X M E S O G N A T H I C D R I F T
R R A E V V C E I U P M T E R M I N A L
H C E O M L E E W A Y D E V I A T I O N
D L P T M A P A R A F U N C T I O N A L
E E B R R X T T O V E R B I T E S T E P
P N A S O O Z U C R O S S B I T E O T J
R C L B C T G Q R T F O C C L U S I O N
E H A R T E R N C E R V I C A L S P E E
S I N U R G N U A V A B F R A C T I O N
S N C X A R D T S T S U P P O R T I N G
I G I I U O I X R I H H S Y N O V I A L
O H N S M U S D Y I O I X O V E R J E T
N W G M A P C Q L I C N C C A P S U L E
```

Introduction

Tooth-drawing assignments emphasize fundamental principles in tooth design, which later have direct practical application in clinical coursework of a student dental professional. It is understood that these initial drawings are most likely to be the student's first attempts at capturing any tooth likeness; therefore, the overriding goal is only to encourage accuracy and discernment of the important features of the teeth and hopefully facilitate the recognition of these tooth details. *Thus any overwhelming artistic inclinations are not what is being exercised with these basic technical drawings of the teeth.*

It is important to also note that these drawings are only two-dimensional and are somewhat limited to fundamental outlines and proportions; real specimens in patients' mouths vary considerably. However, these drawings will serve to help create mental pictures of teeth in their ideal and composite state using each standard view of the individual tooth.

Directions

Step 1. Locate the two blank gridded worksheets in the workbook. Any additional gridded worksheets can be easily scanned and printed for the correct spacing of the grid needed. Correctly label the worksheet at the bottom of the page with the tooth that will be drawn as shown in the smaller professionally drawn figures.

Step 2. Using the attached table of tooth measurements (also included in the associated textbook's Appendix C on tooth measurements), mark off the overall peripheral tooth measurements for each of the gridded view boxes of the tooth. Note that the grid of the blank worksheet is larger than that shown with the professionally drawn tooth outlines to better enable the student to have room to work. Each square of grid equates to 1 mm of actual dimension, so count off as many squares for each peripheral measurement (such as the mesiodistal diameter) as indicated from the table onto the proper area of the gridded worksheet.

Step 3. To establish crown and root proportions, divide each gridded view box into two parts corresponding to these two measurements, except for the incisal or occlusal view.

Step 4. To indicate the height of contour, locate the approximate area of contact between the adjacent teeth and the area of greatest convexity on the labial or buccal, lingual, mesial, and distal surfaces (as mentioned in the associated textbook's Unit 3 on dental anatomy).

Step 5. To locate the root axis line (RAL), draw a line that exactly bisects the overall gridded box showing the overall crown and root measurements. The cementoenamel junction (CEJ) will then be bisected by the RAL. The root apex may or may not be located on this RAL, depending on the tooth's apex traits.

Step 6. To locate the center of the cingulum, midpoint of the incisal ridge, the center of the occlusal table, root apex, or other important feature, divide the crown and root (if included in that particular view box) into imaginary thirds. Then place the cingulum, incisal ridge, occlusal table, or root apex into proper perspective with respect to the other peripheral overall tooth measurements such as the mesiodistal diameter.

Step 7. To complete the crown outline, connect the heights of contour to the incisal ridge or occlusal table, to the CEJ, and to the other heights of contour. Any additional anatomic features such as marginal ridges, depressions, and so forth, can be indicated upon completion of the crown outline.

Step 8. To complete the root outline, follow the directions for developing the crown outline with the understanding that the cervical one third to one half of the root width generally approximates the cervical width of the crown before it starts to narrow considerably to form the root apex.

Step 9. Shading or stippling of the features may now be added, if desired.

Step 10. A drawing evaluation checklist is also included and can be used by both the student and instructor. Multiple copies of the form may be scanned and printed if needed.

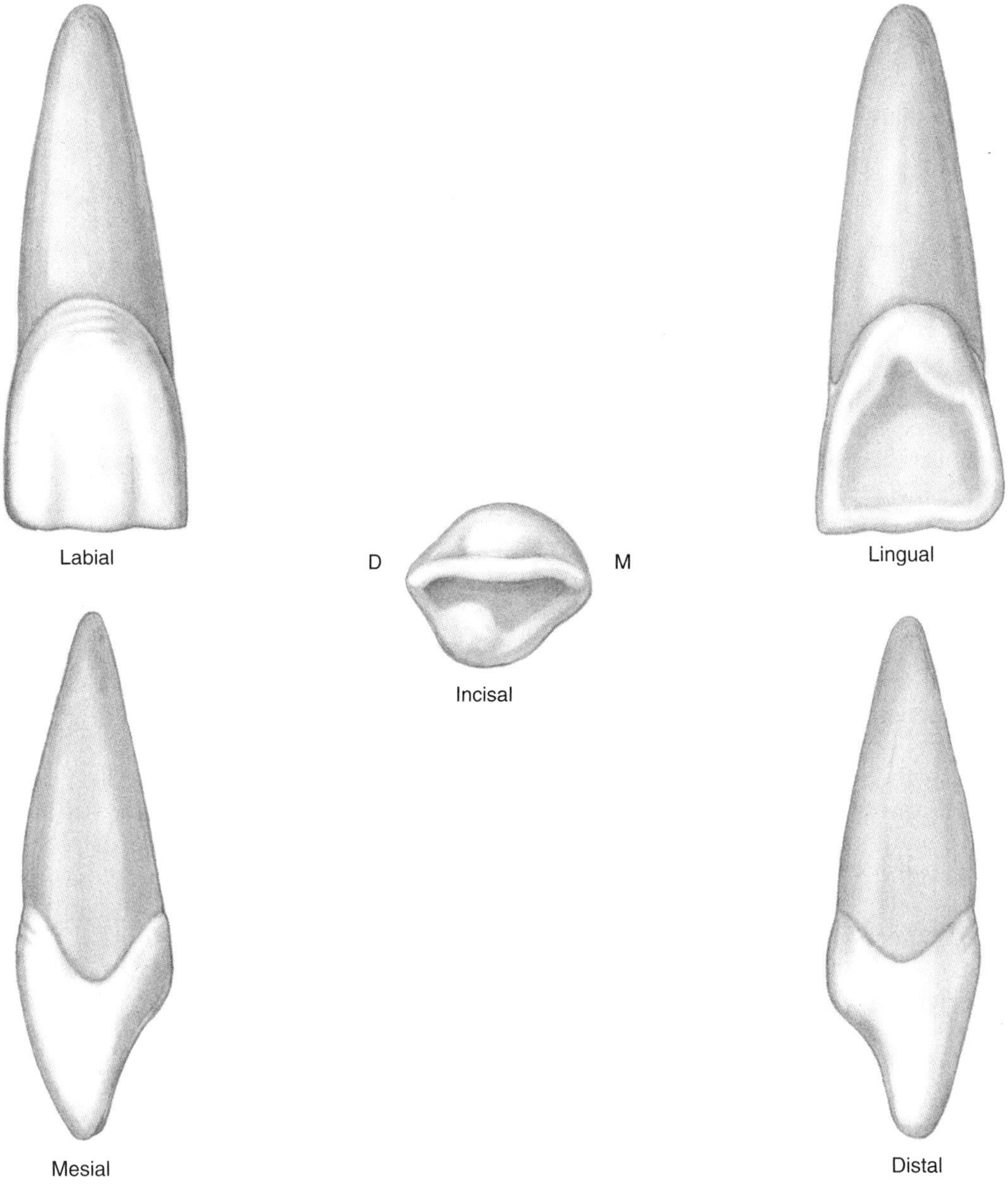

Labial

Lingual

D   M

Incisal

Mesial

Distal

Views of a Permanent Maxillary Right Central Incisor

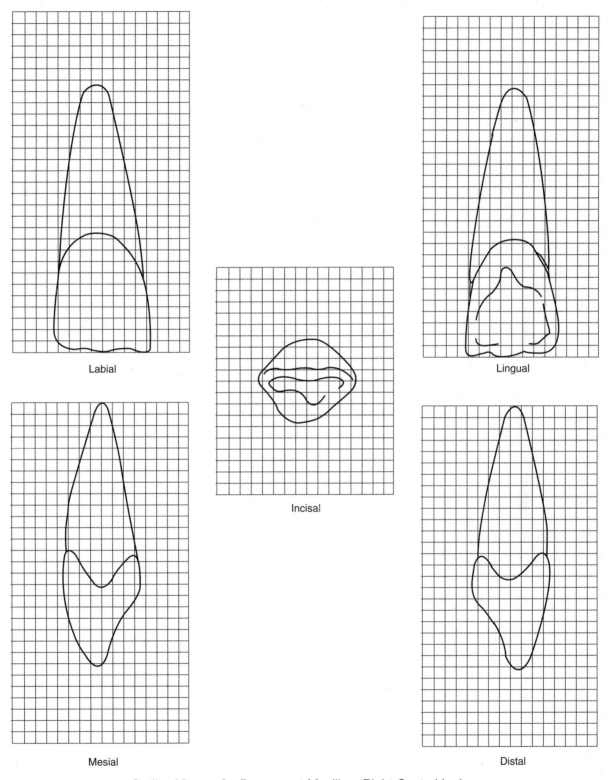

Labial

Incisal

Lingual

Mesial

Distal

Outline Views of a Permanent Maxillary Right Central Incisor

MEASUREMENTS FOR PERMANENT MAXILLARY CENTRAL INCISOR*	
Cervico-Incisal Length of Crown	10.5
Length of Root	13.0
Mesiodistal Diameter of Crown	8.5
Mesiodistal Diameter of CEJ	7.0
Labiolingual Diameter	7.0
Labiolingual Diameter of CEJ	6.0
Curvature of CEJ—Mesial	3.5
Curvature of CEJ—Distal	2.5

*In millimeters; adapted from Nelson SJ: *Wheeler's Dental Anatomy, Physiology, and Occlusions*, ed 9, WB Saunders, Philadelphia, 2009.

CHECKLIST FOR PERMANENT MAXILLARY CENTRAL INCISOR	
Features Noted	**Features Present**
Crown Features	
Incisal ridge, incisal angles, cingulum, marginal ridges, and lingual fossa	
Pronounced distal offset cingulum and marginal ridges, with wide and deep lingual fossa	
Sharper mesioincisal angle and rounder distoincisal angle, with more pronounced mesial CEJ curvature	
Height of contour in cervical third	
Mesial contact is at the incisal third	
Distal contact is at junction of incisal and middle thirds	
Root Features	
Single root	
Overall conical shape, with no proximal root concavities and rounded apex	

Name _____   Tooth Number/Name _____

Date _____   Instructor Rating _____

DRAWING EVALUATION CHECKLIST

RATING SCALE

Completely Correct = 2 points   Major Error = 0 points

Minor Error = 1 point   Note = NA (non-appropriate)

SELF-EVALUATION RATING

Five Views	Clearly Drawn	Accurate Sizing	General Features Included	Specific Features Included
1. Facial View				
2. Lingual View				
3. Mesial View				
4. Distal View				
5. Incisal/ Occlusal View				

Self-Evaluation Rating $= \dfrac{\text{Points received}}{\text{Points possible}} =$ _____ $=$ _____ %

INSTRUCTOR EVALUATION RATING

Five Views	Clearly Drawn	Accurate Sizing	General Features Included	Specific Features Included
1. Facial View				
2. Lingual View				
3. Mesial View				
4. Distal View				
5. Incisal/ Occlusal View				

Instructor Evaluation Rating $= \dfrac{\text{Points received}}{\text{Points possible}} =$ _____ $=$ _____ %

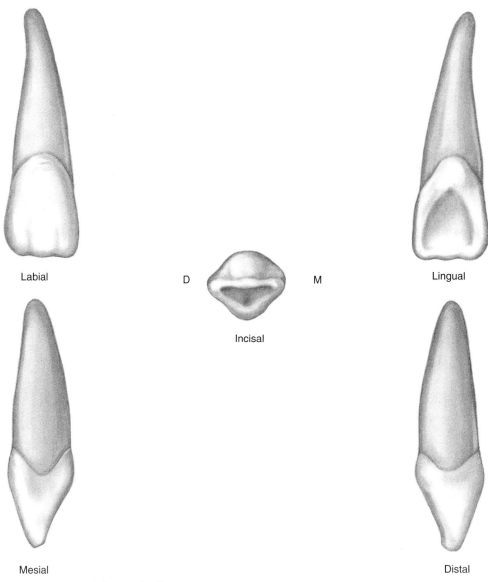

Labial

D   M

Lingual

Incisal

Mesial

Distal

Views of a Permanent Maxillary Right Lateral Incisor

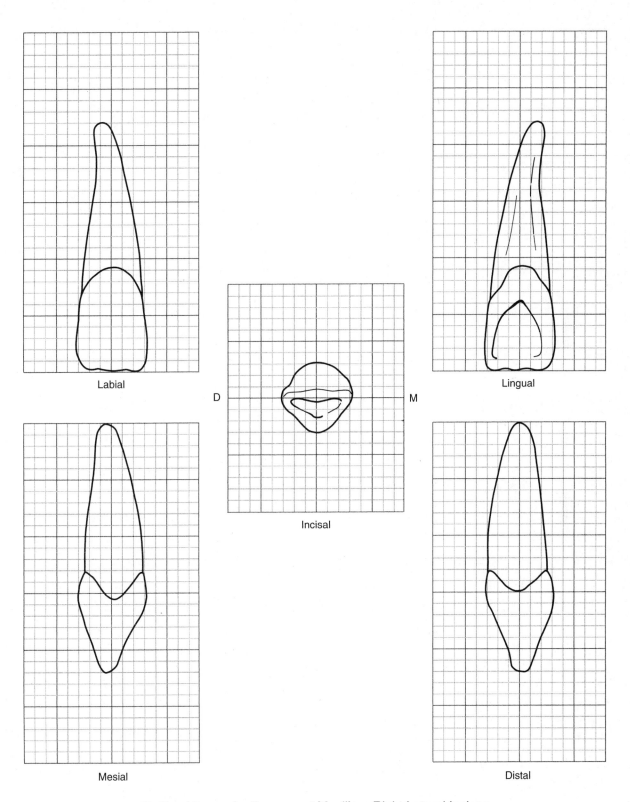

Labial

Lingual

Incisal

Mesial

Distal

Outline Views of a Permanent Maxillary Right Lateral Incisor

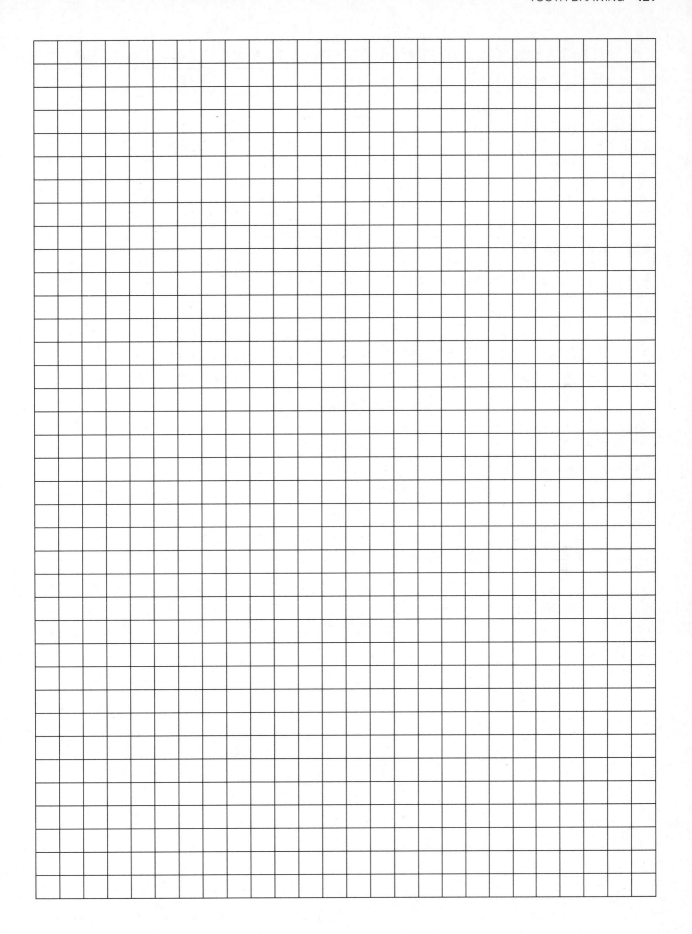

MEASUREMENTS FOR PERMANENT MAXILLARY LATERAL INCISOR*

Cervico-Incisal Length of Crown	9.0
Length of Root	13.0
Mesiodistal Diameter of Crown	6.5
Mesiodistal Diameter of CEJ	5.0
Labiolingual Diameter	6.0
Labiolingual Diameter of CEJ	5.0
Curvature of CEJ—Mesial	3.0
Curvature of CEJ—Distal	2.0

*In millimeters; adapted from Nelson SJ: *Wheeler's Dental Anatomy, Physiology, and Occlusions*, ed 9, WB Saunders, Philadelphia, 2009.

CHECKLIST FOR PERMANENT MAXILLARY LATERAL INCISOR

Features Noted	Features Present
Crown Features	
Incisal ridge, incisal angles, cingulum, marginal ridges, and lingual fossa	
Pronounced lingual surface, with centered cingulum and prominent marginal ridges	
Sharper mesioincisal angle and rounder distoincisal angle, with more pronounced mesial CEJ curvature	
Height of contour in cervical third	
Mesial contact is at incisal third	
Distal contact is at middle third	
Root Features	
Single root	
Overall conical shape, with no proximal root concavities and root curves distally, with sharp apex	

Name _____ Tooth Number/Name _____
Date _____ Instructor Rating _____

DRAWING EVALUATION CHECKLIST

RATING SCALE

Completely Correct = 2 points   Major Error = 0 points
Minor Error = 1 point   Note: NA (non-appropriate)

SELF-EVALUATION RATING

Five Views	Clearly Drawn	Accurate Sizing	General Features Included	Specific Features Included
1. Facial View				
2. Lingual View				
3. Mesial View				
4. Distal View				
5. Incisal/ Occlusal View				

$$\text{Self-Evaluation Rating} = \frac{\text{Points received}}{\text{Points possible}} = \rule{3cm}{0.4pt} = \rule{3cm}{0.4pt}\ \%$$

INSTRUCTOR EVALUATION RATING

Five Views	Clearly Drawn	Accurate Sizing	General Features Included	Specific Features Included
1. Facial View				
2. Lingual View				
3. Mesial View				
4. Distal View				
5. Incisal/ Occlusal View				

$$\text{Instructor Evaluation Rating} = \frac{\text{Points received}}{\text{Points possible}} = \rule{3cm}{0.4pt} = \rule{3cm}{0.4pt}\ \%$$

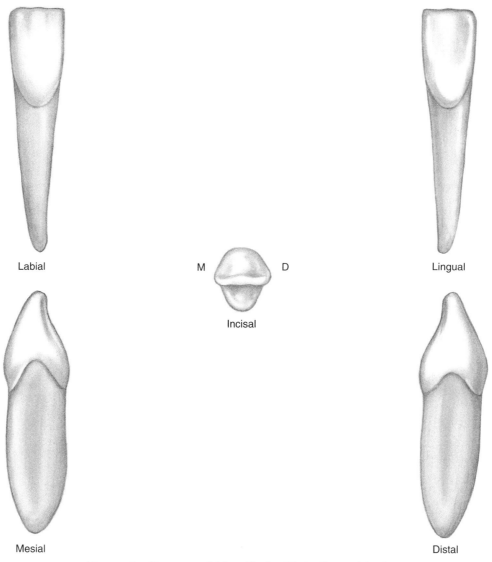

Labial

M D

Incisal

Lingual

Mesial

Distal

Views of a Permanent Mandibular Right Central Incisor

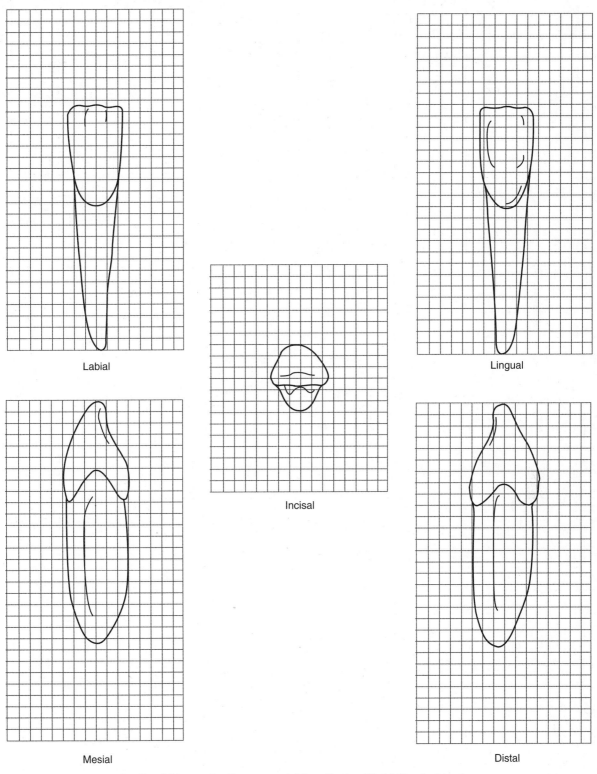

Labial

Lingual

Incisal

Mesial

Distal

Outline Views of a Permanent Mandibular Right Central Incisor

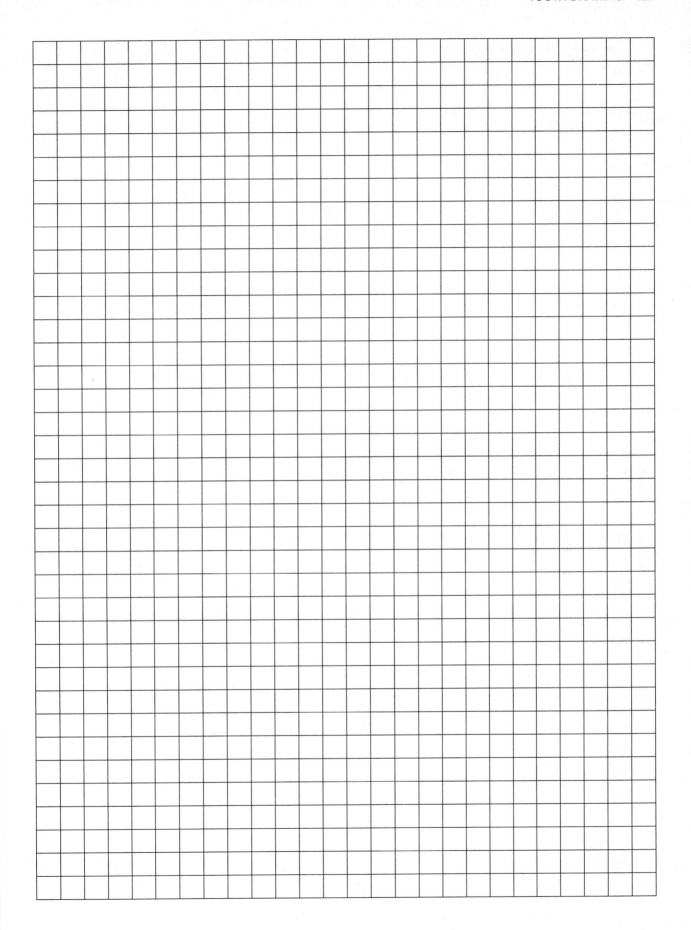

MEASUREMENTS FOR PERMANENT MANDIBULAR CENTRAL INCISOR*

Cervico-Incisal Length of Crown	9.0
Length of Root	12.5
Mesiodistal Diameter of Crown	5.0
Mesiodistal Diameter of CEJ	3.5
Labiolingual Diameter	6.0
Labiolingual Diameter of CEJ	5.3
Curvature of CEJ—Mesial	3.0
Curvature of CEJ—Distal	2.0

*In millimeters; adapted from Nelson SJ: *Wheeler's Dental Anatomy, Physiology, and Occlusions*, ed 9, WB Saunders, Philadelphia, 2009.

CHECKLIST FOR PERMANENT MANDIBULAR CENTRAL INCISOR

Features Noted	Features Present
Crown Features	
Incisal ridge, incisal angles, cingulum, marginal ridges, and lingual fossa	
Symmetric, with small centered cingulum and less pronounced marginal ridges and lingual fossa	
Sharper mesioincisal angle and rounder distoincisal angle, with more pronounced mesial CEJ curvature	
Height of contour in cervical third	
Mesial contact is at incisal third	
Distal contact is at incisal third	
Root Features	
Single root	
Root is longer than the crown and pronounced proximal root concavities	

Name _____   Tooth Number/Name _____

Date _____   Instructor Rating _____

DRAWING EVALUATION CHECKLIST

RATING SCALE

Completely Correct = 2 points   Major Error = 0 points

Minor Error = 1 point   Note: NA (non-appropriate)

SELF-EVALUATION RATING

Five Views	Clearly Drawn	Accurate Sizing	General Features Included	Specific Features Included
1. Facial View				
2. Lingual View				
3. Mesial View				
4. Distal View				
5. Incisal/ Occlusal View				

Self-Evaluation Rating = $\dfrac{\text{Points received}}{\text{Points possible}}$ = _____ = _____ %

INSTRUCTOR EVALUATION RATING

Five Views	Clearly Drawn	Accurate Sizing	General Features Included	Specific Features Included
1. Facial View				
2. Lingual View				
3. Mesial View				
4. Distal View				
5. Incisal/ Occlusal View				

Instructor Evaluation Rating = $\dfrac{\text{Points received}}{\text{Points possible}}$ = _____ = _____ %

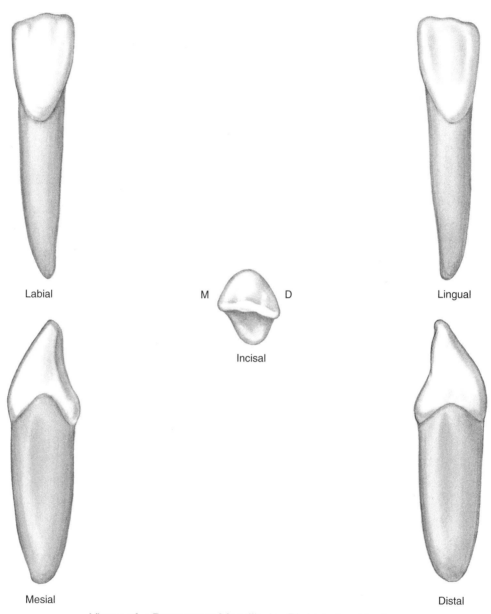

Labial

Lingual

M ◯ D

Incisal

Mesial

Distal

Views of a Permanent Mandibular Right Lateral Incisor

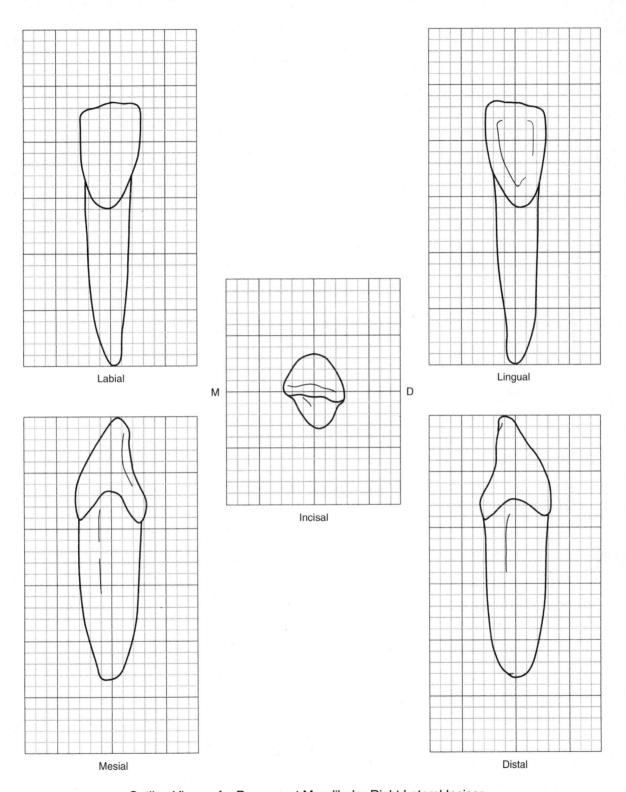

Labial

Lingual

M

D

Incisal

Mesial

Distal

Outline Views of a Permanent Mandibular Right Lateral Incisor

MEASUREMENTS FOR PERMANENT MANDIBULAR LATERAL INCISOR*	
Cervico-Incisal Length of Crown	9.5
Length of Root	14.0
Mesiodistal Diameter of Crown	5.5
Mesiodistal Diameter of CEJ	4.0
Labiolingual Diameter	6.5
Labiolingual Diameter of CEJ	5.8
Curvature of CEJ—Mesial	3.0
Curvature of CEJ—Distal	2.0

*In millimeters; adapted from Nelson SJ. *Wheeler's Dental Anatomy, Physiology, and Occlusions*, ed 9. Saunders, Philadelphia, 2009.

CHECKLIST FOR PERMANENT MANDIBULAR LATERAL INCISOR	
Features Noted	**Features Present**
Crown Features	
Incisal ridge, incisal angles, cingulum, marginal ridges, and lingual fossa	
Not symmetric and appears twisted distally	
Small, distally placed cingulum, with mesial marginal ridge longer than distal marginal ridge	
Sharper mesioincisal angle and rounder distoincisal angle, with more pronounced mesial CEJ curvature	
Height of contour in cervical third	
Mesial contact is at incisal third	
Distal contact is at incisal third	
Root Features	
Single root	
Root is longer than the crown and proximal root concavities	

Name _____   Tooth Number/Name _____

Date _____   Instructor Rating _____

DRAWING EVALUATION CHECKLIST

RATING SCALE
Completely Correct = 2 points   Major Error = 0 points

Minor Error = 1 point   Note: NA (non-appropriate)

SELF-EVALUATION RATING

Five Views	Clearly Drawn	Accurate Sizing	General Features Included	Specific Features Included
1. Facial View				
2. Lingual View				
3. Mesial View				
4. Distal View				
5. Incisal/ Occlusal View				

Self-Evaluation Rating $= \dfrac{\text{Points received}}{\text{Points possible}} =$ _____ $=$ _____ %

INSTRUCTOR EVALUATION RATING

Five Views	Clearly Drawn	Accurate Sizing	General Features Included	Specific Features Included
1. Facial View				
2. Lingual View				
3. Mesial View				
4. Distal View				
5. Incisal/ Occlusal View				

Instructor Evaluation Rating $= \dfrac{\text{Points received}}{\text{Points possible}} =$ _____ $=$ _____ %

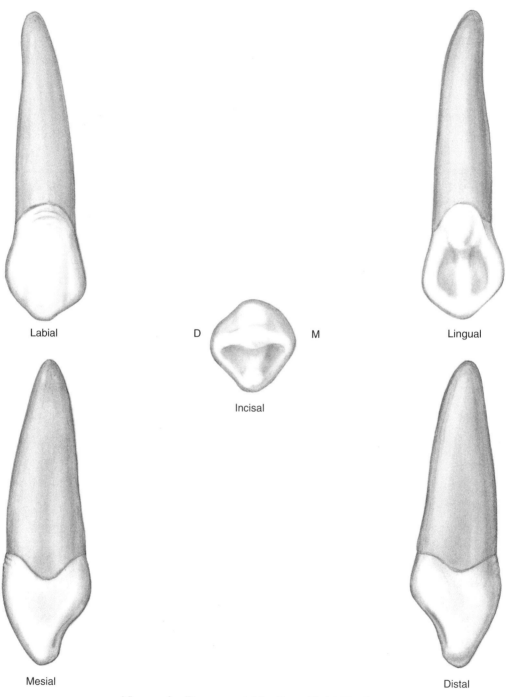

Labial

D   M

Incisal

Lingual

Mesial

Distal

Views of a Permanent Maxillary Right Canine

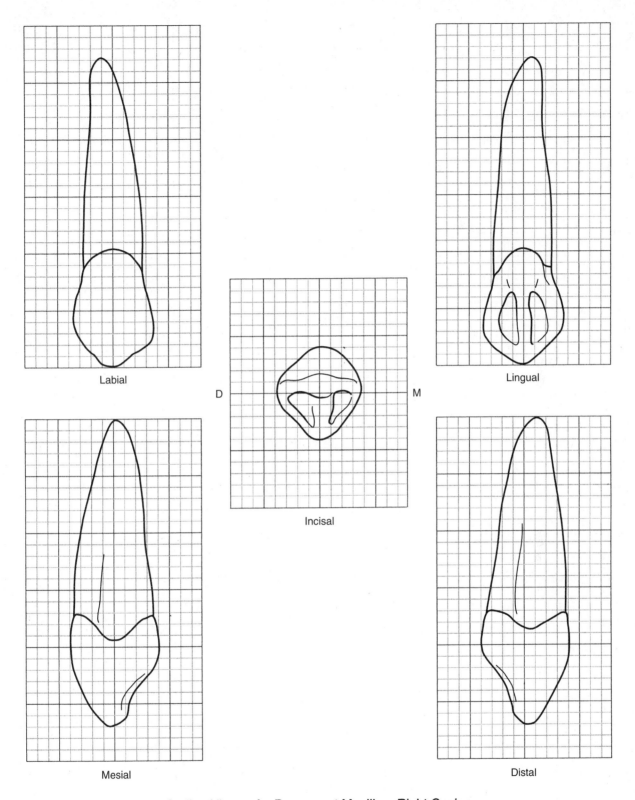

Labial

Lingual

D

M

Incisal

Mesial

Distal

Outline Views of a Permanent Maxillary Right Canine

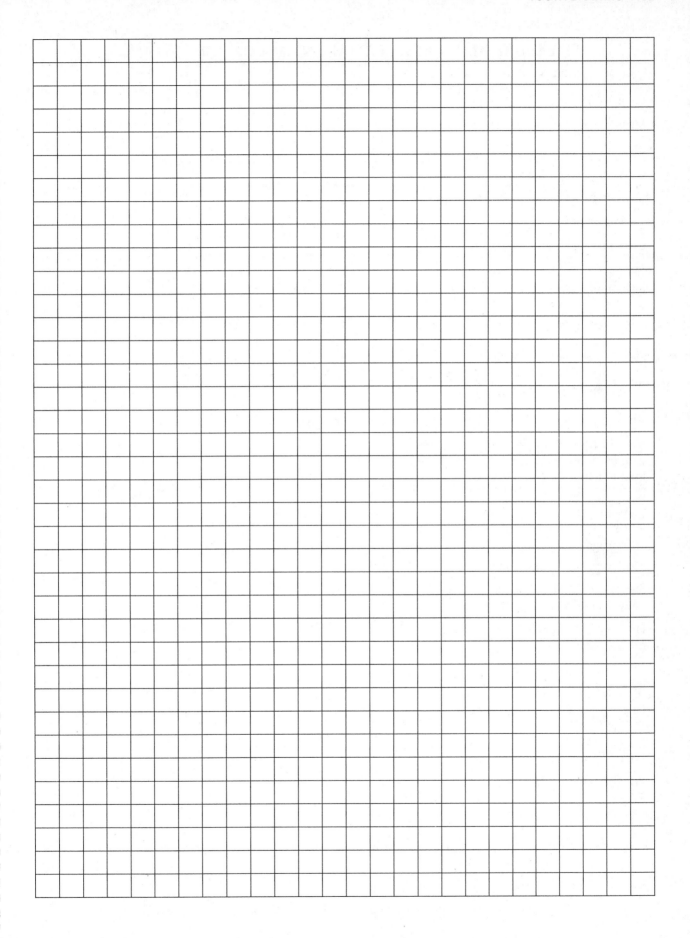

MEASUREMENTS FOR PERMANENT MAXILLARY CANINE*	
Cervico-Incisal Length of Crown	10.0
Length of Root	17.0
Mesiodistal Diameter of Crown	7.5
Mesiodistal Diameter of CEJ	5.5
Labiolingual Diameter	8.0
Labiolingual Diameter of CEJ	7.0
Curvature of CEJ—Mesial	2.5
Curvature of CEJ—Distal	1.5

*In millimeters; adapted from Nelson SJ: *Wheeler's Dental Anatomy, Physiology, and Occlusions*, ed 9, WB Saunders, Philadelphia, 2009.

CHECKLIST FOR PERMANENT MAXILLARY CANINE	
Features Noted	**Features Present**
Crown Features	
Single cusp with tip and slopes, labial ridge, cingulum, lingual ridge, marginal ridges, and lingual fossae	
Prominent lingual surface, with sharp cusp tip	
Shorter mesial cusp slope, with more pronounced mesial CEJ curvature	
More cervical contact on distal	
Shorter distal outline on labial view with depression between the distal contact and CEJ	
Height of contour for labial is cervical third and for lingual is middle third	
Mesial contact is at junction of incisal third and middle thirds	
Distal contact is at middle third	
Root Features	
Long, thick single root	
Proximal root concavities and blunt root apex	

Name _____   Tooth Number/Name _____

Date _____   Instructor Rating _____

DRAWING EVALUATION CHECKLIST

RATING SCALE

Completely Correct = 2 points   Major Error = 0 points

Minor Error = 1 point   Note: NA (non-appropriate)

SELF-EVALUATION RATING

Five Views	Clearly Drawn	Accurate Sizing	General Features Included	Specific Features Included
1. Facial View				
2. Lingual View				
3. Mesial View				
4. Distal View				
5. Incisal/ Occlusal View				

Self-Evaluation Rating = $\dfrac{\text{Points received}}{\text{Points possible}}$ = _____ = _____ %

INSTRUCTOR EVALUATION RATING

Five Views	Clearly Drawn	Accurate Sizing	General Features Included	Specific Features Included
1. Facial View				
2. Lingual View				
3. Mesial View				
4. Distal View				
5. Incisal/ Occlusal View				

Instructor Evaluation Rating = $\dfrac{\text{Points received}}{\text{Points possible}}$ = _____ = _____ %

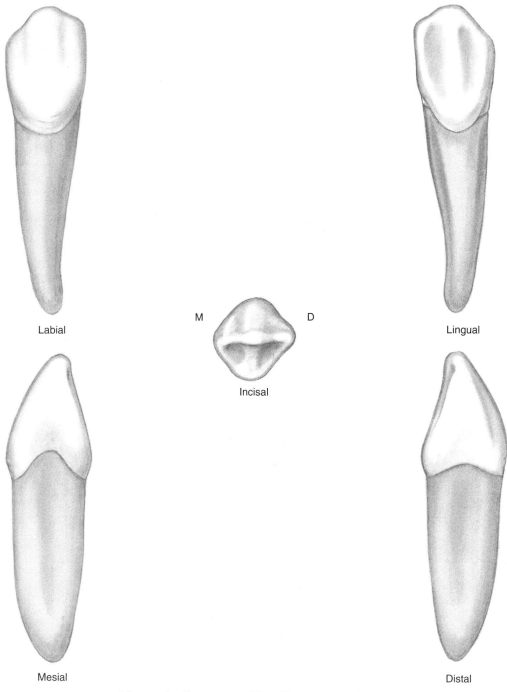

Labial

M   D

Incisal

Lingual

Mesial

Distal

Views of a Permanent Mandibular Right Canine

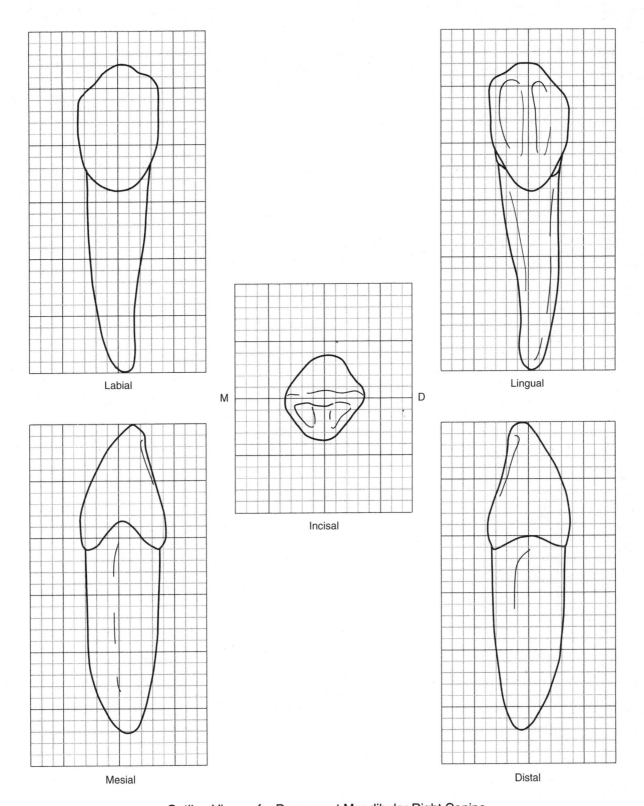

Labial

Lingual

M

D

Incisal

Mesial

Distal

Outline Views of a Permanent Mandibular Right Canine

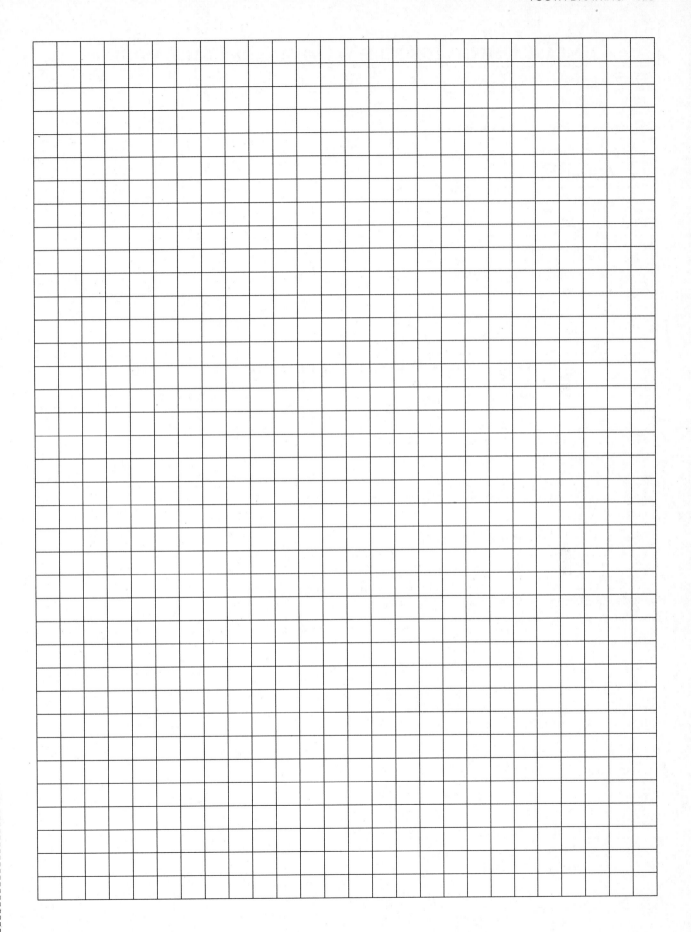

MEASUREMENTS FOR PERMANENT MANDIBULAR CANINE*	
Cervico-Incisal Length of Crown	11.0
Length of Root	16.0
Mesiodistal Diameter of Crown	7.0
Mesiodistal Diameter of CEJ	5.5
Labiolingual Diameter	7.5
Labiolingual Diameter of CEJ	7.0
Curvature of CEJ—Mesial	2.5
Curvature of CEJ—Distal	1.0

*In millimeters; adapted from Nelson SJ: *Wheeler's Dental Anatomy, Physiology, and Occlusions*, ed 9, WB Saunders, Philadelphia, 2009.

CHECKLIST FOR PERMANENT MANDIBULAR CANINE	
Features Noted	**Features Present**
Crown Features	
Single cusp with tip and slopes, labial ridge, cingulum, lingual ridge, marginal ridges, and lingual fossae	
Less pronounced lingual surface, with less sharp cusp tip	
Shorter mesial cusp slope, with more pronounced mesial CEJ curvature	
More cervical contact on distal	
Shorter and rounder distal outline on labial view, with a shorter mesial slope than distal	
Height of contour for labial is cervical third and for lingual is middle third	
Mesial contact is at incisal third	
Distal contact is at junction of incisal and middle thirds	
Root Features	
Long, thick single root	
Proximal root concavities, with developmental depressions on mesial and distal giving tooth double-rooted appearance, and pointed apex	

Name _____   Tooth Number/Name _____

Date _____   Instructor Rating _____

DRAWING EVALUATION CHECKLIST

RATING SCALE

Completely Correct = 2 points   Major Error = 0 points

Minor Error = 1 point   Note: NA (non-appropriate)

SELF-EVALUATION RATING

Five Views	Clearly Drawn	Accurate Sizing	General Features Included	Specific Features Included
1. Facial View				
2. Lingual View				
3. Mesial View				
4. Distal View				
5. Incisal/ Occlusal View				

Self-Evaluation Rating $= \dfrac{\text{Points received}}{\text{Points possible}} =$ _____ $=$ _____ %

INSTRUCTOR EVALUATION RATING

Five Views	Clearly Drawn	Accurate Sizing	General Features Included	Specific Features Included
1. Facial View				
2. Lingual View				
3. Mesial View				
4. Distal View				
5. Incisal/ Occlusal View				

Instructor Evaluation Rating $= \dfrac{\text{Points received}}{\text{Points possible}} =$ _____ $=$ _____ %

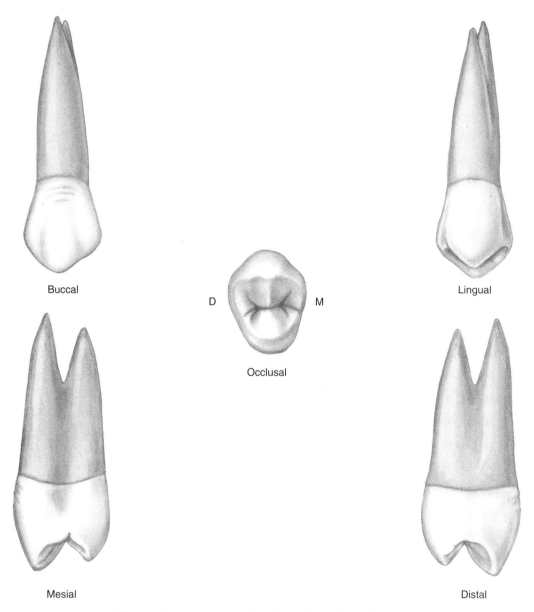

Buccal

D M

Occlusal

Lingual

Mesial

Distal

Views of a Permanent Maxillary Right First Premolar

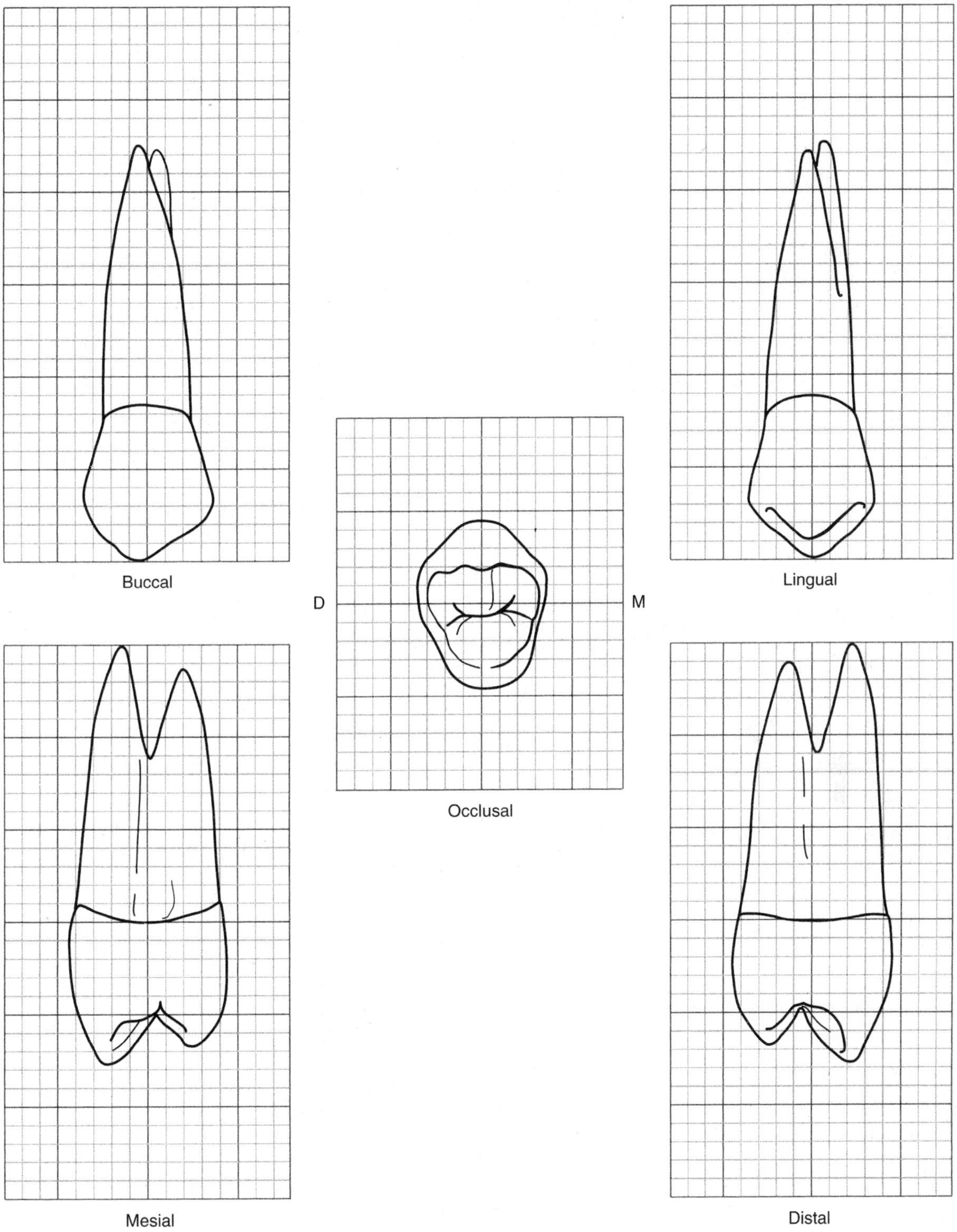

Buccal

Lingual

D

M

Occlusal

Mesial

Distal

Outline Views of a Permanent Maxillary Right First Premolar

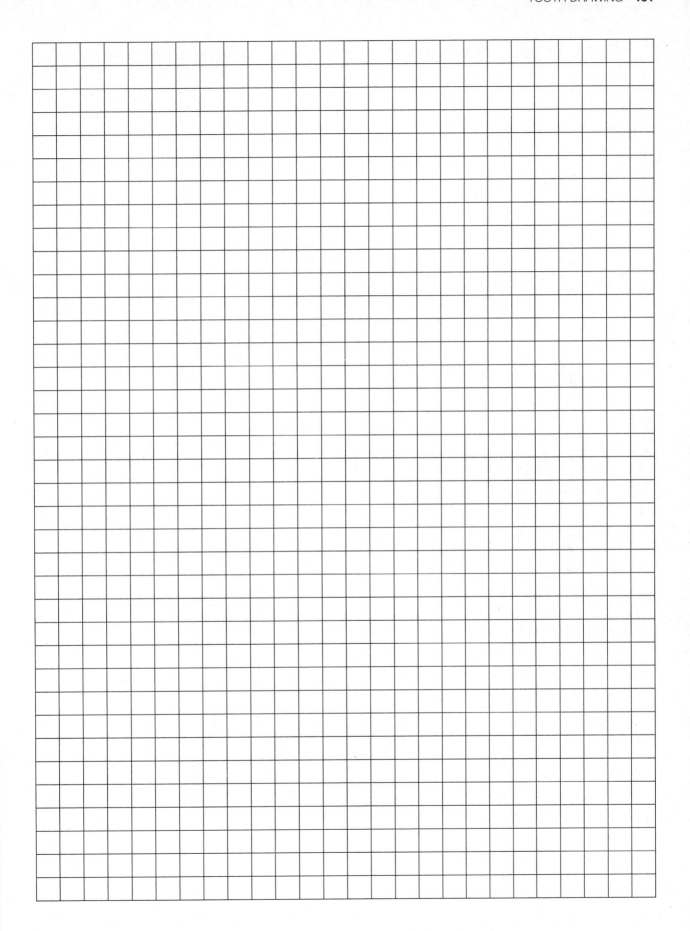

MEASUREMENTS FOR PERMANENT MAXILLARY FIRST PREMOLAR*	
Cervico-occlusal Length of Crown	8.5
Length of Root	14.0
Mesiodistal Diameter of Crown	7.0
Mesiodistal Diameter of CEJ	5.0
Buccolingual Diameter	9.0
Buccolingual Diameter of CEJ	8.0
Curvature of CEJ—Mesial	1.0
Curvature of CEJ—Distal	0.0

*In millimeters; adapted from Nelson SJ: *Wheeler's Dental Anatomy, Physiology, and Occlusions*, ed 9, WB Saunders, Philadelphia, 2009.

CHECKLIST FOR PERMANENT MAXILLARY FIRST PREMOLAR	
Features Noted	**Features Present**
Crown Features	
Occlusal table with marginal ridges and cusps with tips, ridges, inclined planes, and grooves	
Buccal cusp longer of two cusps, with long central groove	
Longer mesial cusp slope than distal cusp slope, with mesial features: deeper CEJ curvature, marginal groove, developmental depression	
Buccal ridge	
Height of contour for the buccal is in cervical third and lingual in middle third	
Mesial and distal contact is just cervical to the junction of occlusal and middle thirds	
Root Features	
Two roots with root trunk	
Proximal root concavities	

Name _____   Tooth Number/Name _____

Date _____   Instructor Rating _____

DRAWING EVALUATION CHECKLIST

RATING SCALE

Completely Correct = 2 points   Major Error = 0 points

Minor Error = 1 point   Note: NA (non-appropriate)

SELF-EVALUATION RATING

Five Views	Clearly Drawn	Accurate Sizing	General Features Included	Specific Features Included
1. Facial View				
2. Lingual View				
3. Mesial View				
4. Distal View				
5. Incisal/ Occlusal View				

$$\text{Self-Evaluation Rating} = \frac{\text{Points received}}{\text{Points possible}} = \underline{\hspace{3cm}} = \underline{\hspace{3cm}} \%$$

INSTRUCTOR EVALUATION RATING

Five Views	Clearly Drawn	Accurate Sizing	General Features Included	Specific Features Included
1. Facial View				
2. Lingual View				
3. Mesial View				
4. Distal View				
5. Incisal/ Occlusal View				

$$\text{Instructor Evaluation Rating} = \frac{\text{Points received}}{\text{Points possible}} = \underline{\hspace{3cm}} = \underline{\hspace{3cm}} \%$$

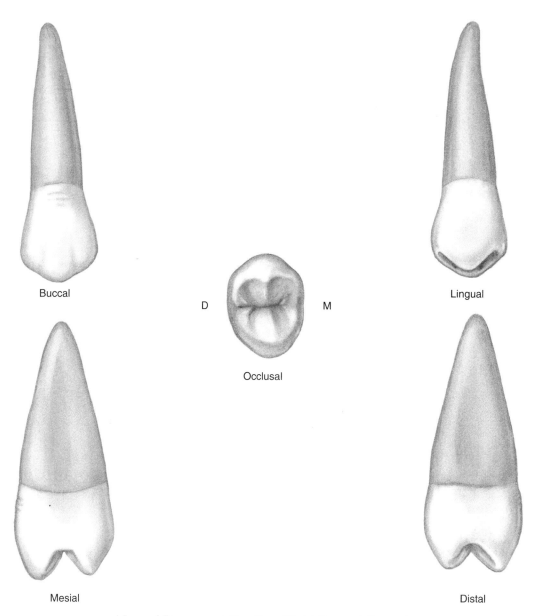

Buccal

Lingual

D   M

Occlusal

Mesial

Distal

View of Permanent Maxillary Right Second Premolar

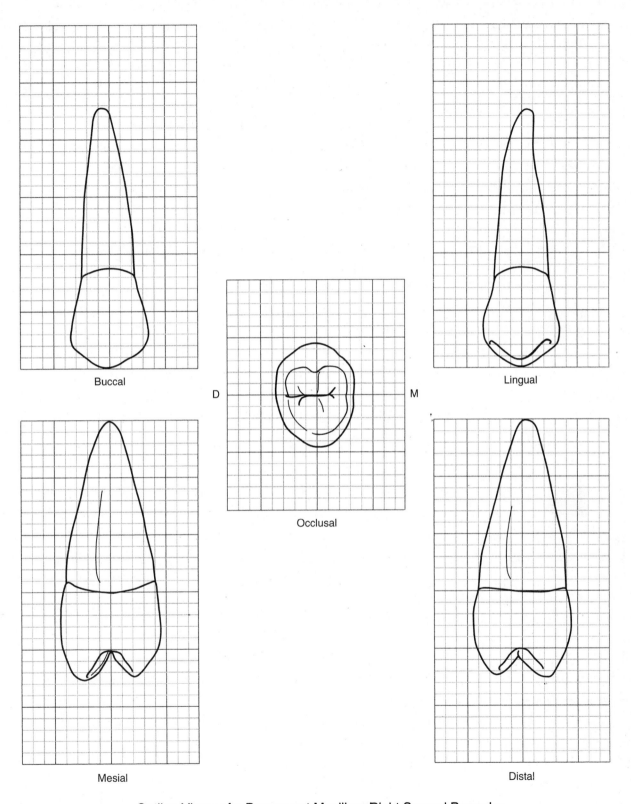

Buccal

Lingual

D   M

Occlusal

Mesial

Distal

Outline Views of a Permanent Maxillary Right Second Premolar

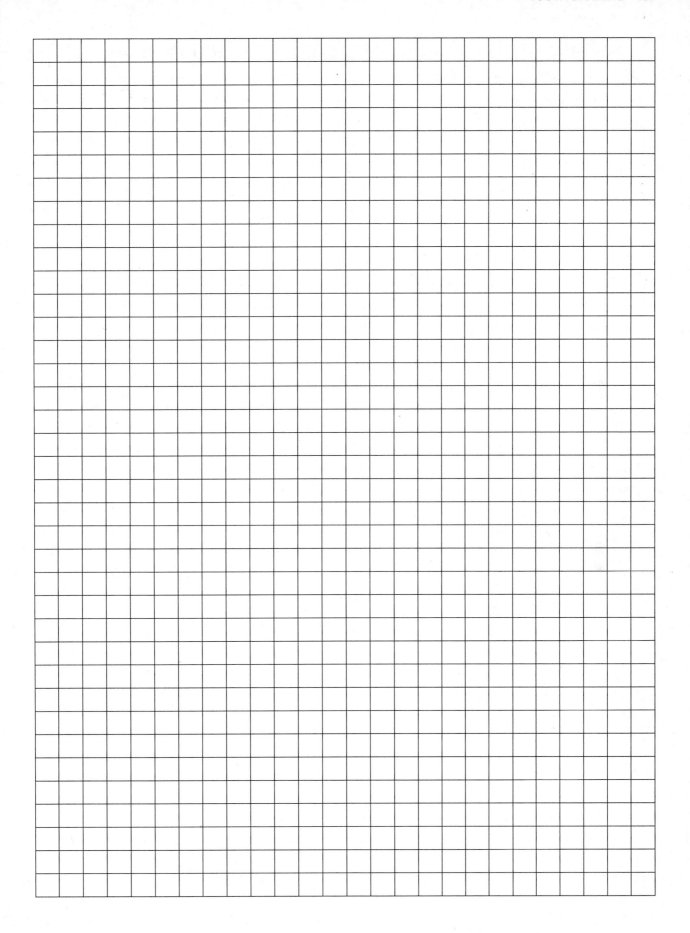

MEASUREMENTS FOR PERMANENT MAXILLARY SECOND PREMOLAR*

Cervico-occlusal Length of Crown	8.5
Length of Root	14.0
Mesiodistal Diameter of Crown	7.0
Mesiodistal Diameter of CEJ	5.0
Buccolingual Diameter	9.0
Buccolingual Diameter of CEJ	8.0
Curvature of CEJ—Mesial	1.0
Curvature of CEJ—Distal	0.0

*In millimeters; adapted from Nelson SJ: *Wheeler's Dental Anatomy, Physiology, and Occlusions*, ed 9, WB Saunders, Philadelphia, 2009.

CHECKLIST FOR PERMANENT MAXILLARY SECOND PREMOLAR

Features Noted	Features Present
Crown Features	
Occlusal table with marginal ridges and cusps with tips, ridges, inclined planes, and grooves fossae, pits	
Two cusps same length, with short central groove	
Lingual cusp offset to the mesial	
Buccal ridge	
Height of contour for the buccal is in cervical third and lingual in middle third	
Mesial and distal contact is just cervical to the junction of occlusal and middle thirds	
Root Features	
Single rooted	
Proximal root concavities	

Name _____   Tooth Number/Name _____
Date _____   Instructor Rating _____

DRAWING EVALUATION CHECKLIST

RATING SCALE
Completely Correct = 2 points   Major Error = 0 points
Minor Error = 1 point   Note: NA (non-appropriate)

SELF-EVALUATION RATING

Five Views	Clearly Drawn	Accurate Sizing	General Features Included	Specific Features Included
1. Facial View				
2. Lingual View				
3. Mesial View				
4. Distal View				
5. Incisal/ Occlusal View				

$$\text{Self-Evaluation Rating} = \frac{\text{Points received}}{\text{Points possible}} = \underline{\hspace{2cm}} = \underline{\hspace{2cm}} \%$$

INSTRUCTOR EVALUATION RATING

Five Views	Clearly Drawn	Accurate Sizing	General Features Included	Specific Features Included
1. Facial View				
2. Lingual View				
3. Mesial View				
4. Distal View				
5. Incisal/ Occlusal View				

$$\text{Instructor Evaluation Rating} = \frac{\text{Points received}}{\text{Points possible}} = \underline{\hspace{2cm}} = \underline{\hspace{2cm}} \%$$

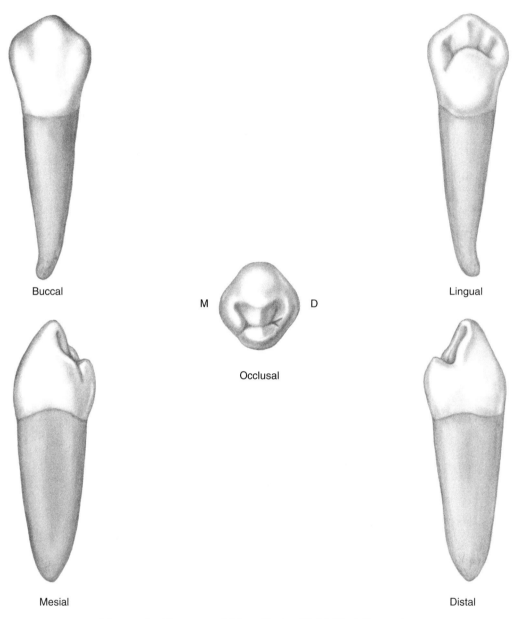

Buccal

Lingual

M   D

Occlusal

Mesial

Distal

Views of a Permanent Mandibular Right First Premolar

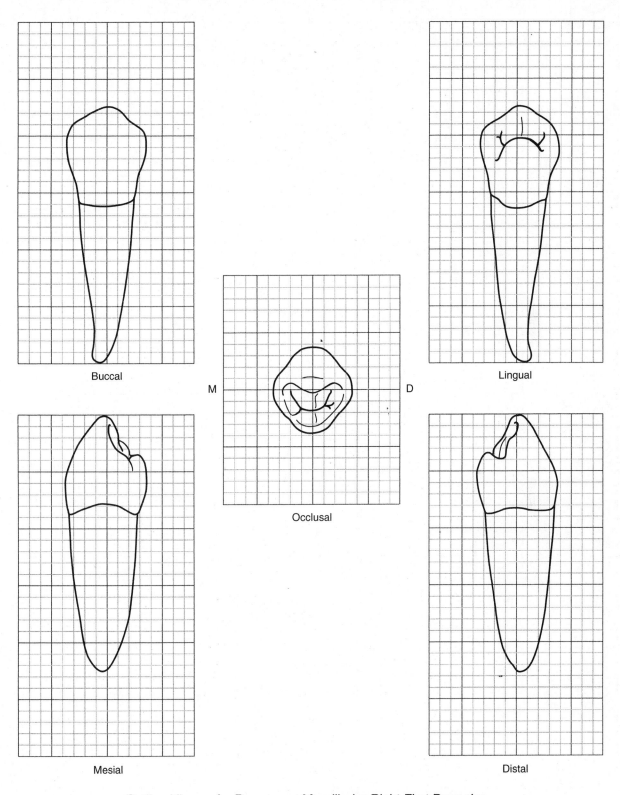

Buccal

Lingual

M

D

Occlusal

Mesial

Distal

Outline Views of a Permanent Mandibular Right First Premolar

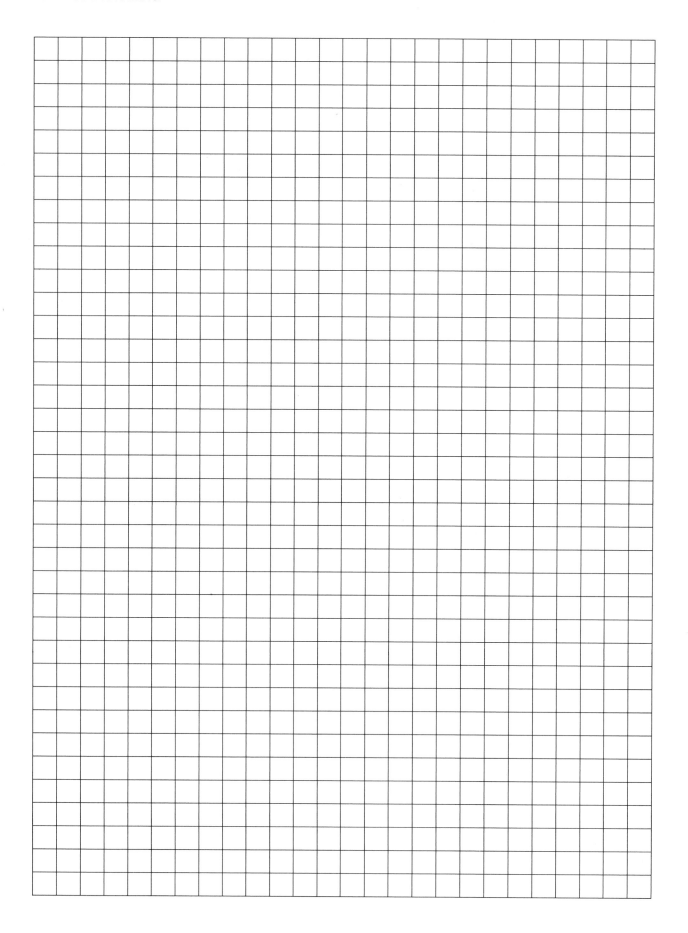

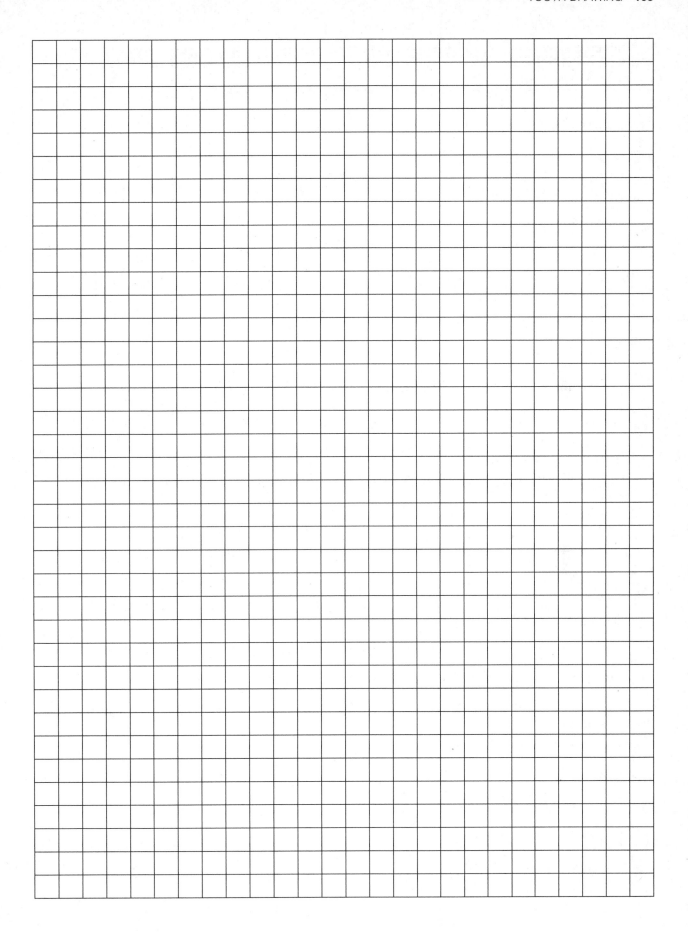

MEASUREMENTS FOR PERMANENT MANDIBULAR FIRST PREMOLAR*	
Cervico-occlusal Length of Crown	8.5
Length of Root	14.0
Mesiodistal Diameter of Crown	7.0
Mesiodistal Diameter of CEJ	5.0
Buccolingual Diameter	7.5
Buccolingual Diameter of CEJ	6.5
Curvature of CEJ—Mesial	1.0
Curvature of CEJ—Distal	0.0

*In millimeters; adapted from Nelson SJ: *Wheeler's Dental Anatomy, Physiology, and Occlusions*, ed 9, WB Saunders, Philadelphia, 2009.

CHECKLIST FOR PERMANENT MANDIBULAR FIRST PREMOLAR	
Features Noted	**Features Present**
Crown Features	
Occlusal table with marginal ridges and cusps with tips, ridges, inclined planes, and grooves, fossae, pits	
Smaller lingual cusp of two cusps	
Shorter mesial cusp slope, with mesial surface features of deeper mesial CEJ curvature and mesiolingual groove	
Buccal ridge	
Height of contour for the buccal is in cervical third and lingual in middle third	
Mesial and distal contact is just cervical to the junction of occlusal and middle thirds	
Root Features	
Single rooted	
Proximal root concavities	

Name _____   Tooth Number/Name _____

Date _____   Instructor Rating _____

DRAWING EVALUATION CHECKLIST

RATING SCALE

Completely Correct = 2 points   Major Error = 0 points

Minor Error = 1 point   Note: NA (non-appropriate)

SELF-EVALUATION RATING

Five Views	Clearly Drawn	Accurate Sizing	General Features Included	Specific Features Included
1. Facial View				
2. Lingual View				
3. Mesial View				
4. Distal View				
5. Incisal/ Occlusal View				

$$\text{Self-Evaluation Rating} = \frac{\text{Points received}}{\text{Points possible}} = \underline{\hspace{2cm}} = \underline{\hspace{2cm}} \%$$

INSTRUCTOR EVALUATION RATING

Five Views	Clearly Drawn	Accurate Sizing	General Features Included	Specific Features Included
1. Facial View				
2. Lingual View				
3. Mesial View				
4. Distal View				
5. Incisal/ Occlusal View				

$$\text{Instructor Evaluation Rating} = \frac{\text{Points received}}{\text{Points possible}} = \underline{\hspace{2cm}} = \underline{\hspace{2cm}} \%$$

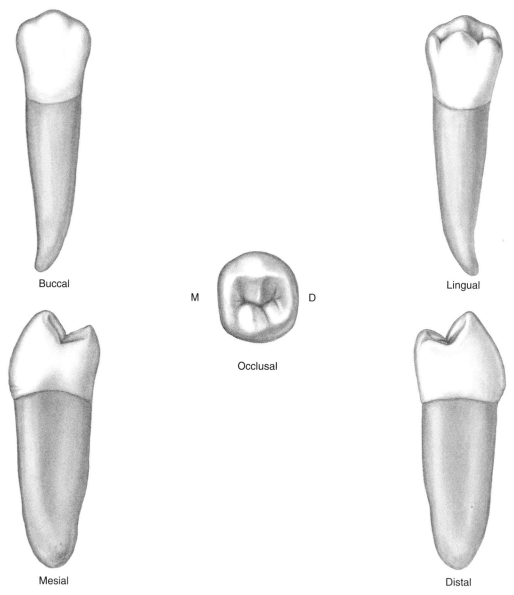

Buccal

Lingual

M   D

Occlusal

Mesial

Distal

Views of a Permanent Mandibular Right Second Premolar (Three-Cusp Type)

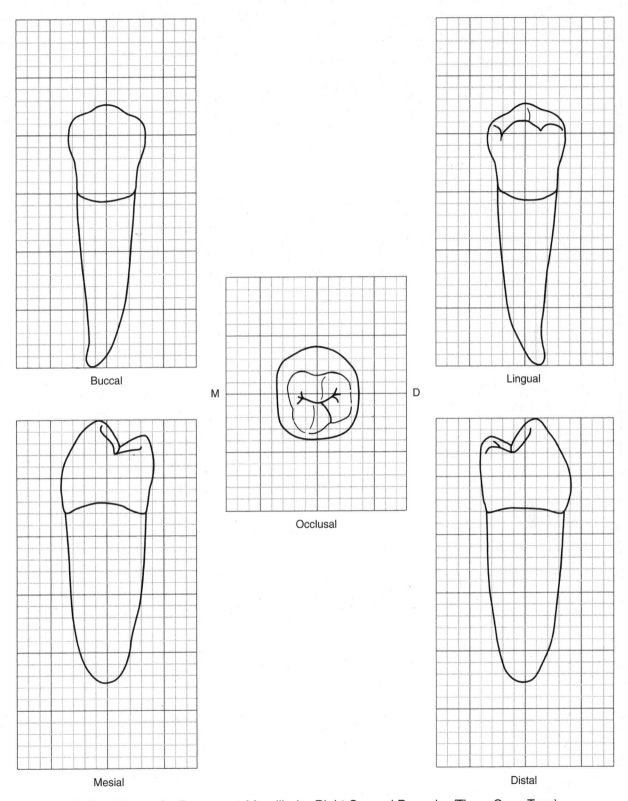

Buccal

Lingual

M   D

Occlusal

Mesial

Distal

Outline Views of a Permanent Mandibular Right Second Premolar (Three-Cusp Type)

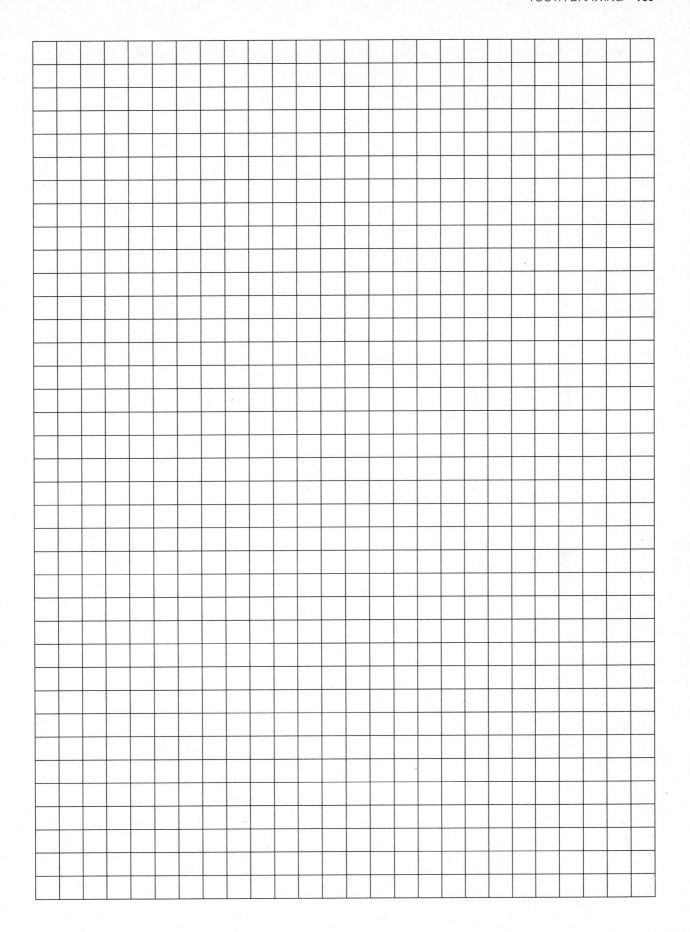

MEASUREMENTS FOR PERMANENT MANDIBULAR SECOND PREMOLAR (Three-Cusp Type) *	
Cervico-occlusal Length of Crown	8.0
Length of Root	14.5
Mesiodistal Diameter of Crown	7.0
Mesiodistal Diameter of CEJ	5.0
Buccolingual Diameter	8.0
Buccolingual Diameter of CEJ	7.0
Curvature of CEJ—Mesial	1.0
Curvature of CEJ—Distal	0.0

*In millimeters; adapted from Nelson SJ: *Wheeler's Dental Anatomy, Physiology, and Occlusions*, ed 9, WB Saunders, Philadelphia, 2009.

CHECKLIST FOR PERMANENT MANDIBULAR SECOND PREMOLAR (Three-Cusp Type)	
Features Noted	**Features Present**
Crown Features	
Occlusal table with marginal ridges and cusps with tips, ridges, inclined planes, and grooves	
Three cusps with Y-shaped groove pattern	
Distal marginal ridge more cervically located, with more occlusal surface visible from distal view	
Buccal ridge	
Height of contour for the buccal is in cervical third and lingual in middle third	
Mesial and distal contact is just cervical to the junction of occlusal and middle thirds	
Root Features	
Single rooted	
Proximal root concavities	

Name _____   Tooth Number/Name _____

Date _____   Instructor Rating _____

DRAWING EVALUATION CHECKLIST

RATING SCALE

Completely Correct = 2 points   Major Error = 0 points

Minor Error = 1 point   Note: NA (non-appropriate)

SELF-EVALUATION RATING

Five Views	Clearly Drawn	Accurate Sizing	General Features Included	Specific Features Included
1. Facial View				
2. Lingual View				
3. Mesial View				
4. Distal View				
5. Incisal/ Occlusal View				

$$\text{Self-Evaluation Rating} = \frac{\text{Points received}}{\text{Points possible}} = \underline{\hspace{2cm}} = \underline{\hspace{2cm}} \%$$

INSTRUCTOR EVALUATION RATING

Five Views	Clearly Drawn	Accurate Sizing	General Features Included	Specific Features Included
1. Facial View				
2. Lingual View				
3. Mesial View				
4. Distal View				
5. Incisal/ Occlusal View				

$$\text{Instructor Evaluation Rating} = \frac{\text{Points received}}{\text{Points possible}} = \underline{\hspace{2cm}} = \underline{\hspace{2cm}} \%$$

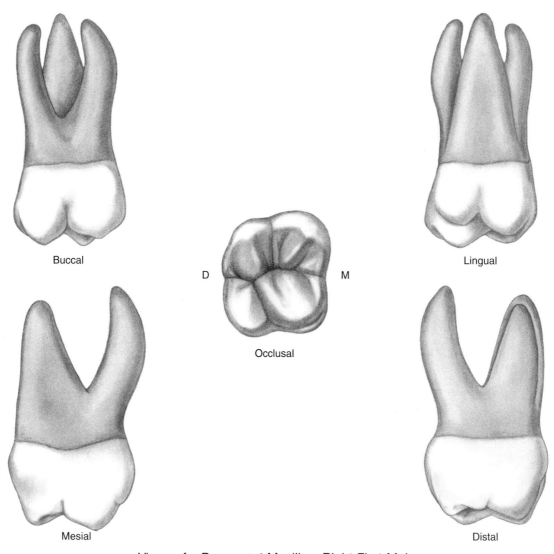

Buccal

Lingual

D   M

Occlusal

Mesial

Distal

Views of a Permanent Maxillary Right First Molar

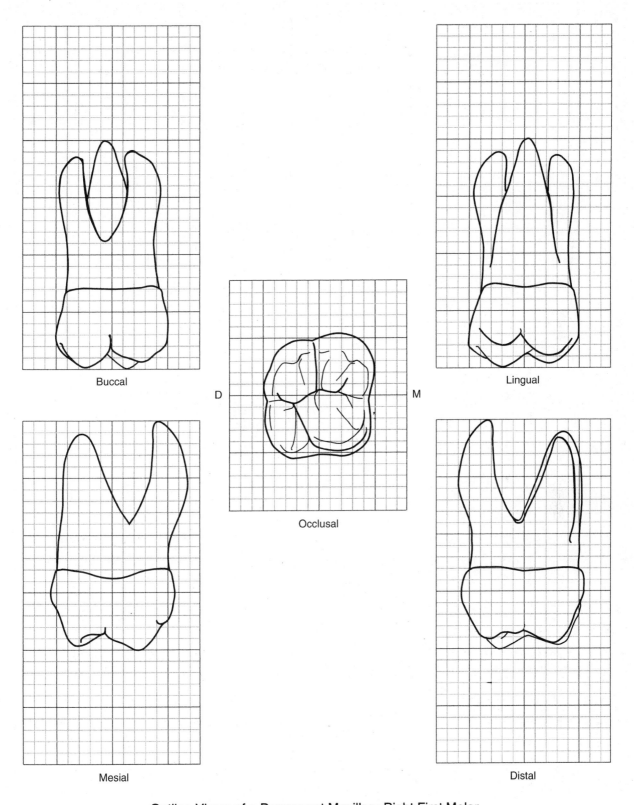

Buccal

Lingual

D   M

Occlusal

Mesial

Distal

Outline Views of a Permanent Maxillary Right First Molar

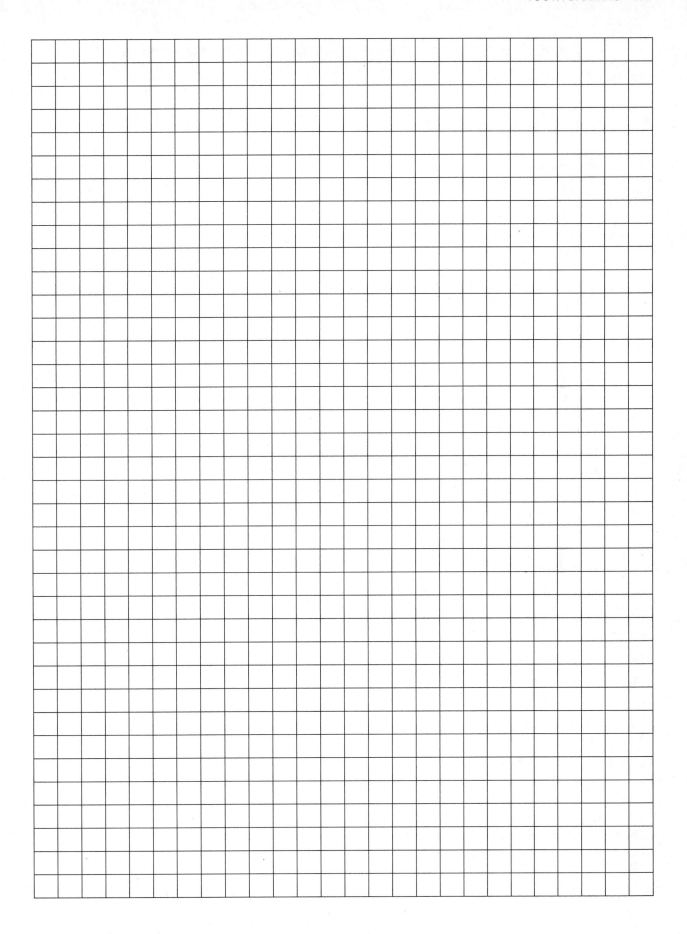

MEASUREMENTS FOR PERMANENT MAXILLARY FIRST MOLAR*	
Cervico-occlusal Length of Crown	7.5
Length of Root	Buccal: 12 Lingual: 13
Mesiodistal Diameter of Crown	10.0
Mesiodistal Diameter of CEJ	8.0
Buccolingual Diameter	11.0
Buccolingual Diameter of CEJ	10.0
Curvature of CEJ—Mesial	1.0
Curvature of CEJ—Distal	0.0

*In millimeters; adapted from Nelson SJ: *Wheeler's Dental Anatomy, Physiology, and Occlusions*, ed 9, WB Saunders, Philadelphia, 2009.

CHECKLIST FOR PERMANENT MAXILLARY FIRST MOLAR	
Features Noted	**Features Present**
Crown Features	
Occlusal table with marginal ridges and cusps with tips, ridges, inclined planes, and grooves, fossae, pits	
Prominent oblique ridge	
Four major cusps with buccal cusps almost equal in height	
Fifth minor cusp of Carabelli associated with mesiolingual cusp and groove	
Mesiolingual cusp outline longer and larger but not as sharp as distolingual cusp outline	
Buccal cervical ridge	
Height of contour for the buccal is in cervical third and lingual in middle third	
Mesial contact is at junction of occlusal and middle thirds	
Distal contact at middle third	
Root Features	
Three roots	
Furcations well removed from CEJ, root trunks, root concavities, and divergent roots	

Name _____   Tooth Number/Name _____

Date _____   Instructor Rating _____

DRAWING EVALUATION CHECKLIST

RATING SCALE

Completely Correct = 2 points   Major Error = 0 points
Minor Error = 1 point   Note: NA (non-appropriate)

SELF-EVALUATION RATING

Five Views	Clearly Drawn	Accurate Sizing	General Features Included	Specific Features Included
1. Facial View				
2. Lingual View				
3. Mesial View				
4. Distal View				
5. Incisal/ Occlusal View				

Self-Evaluation Rating = $\dfrac{\text{Points received}}{\text{Points possible}}$ = _____ = _____ %

INSTRUCTOR EVALUATION RATING

Five Views	Clearly Drawn	Accurate Sizing	General Features Included	Specific Features Included
1. Facial View				
2. Lingual View				
3. Mesial View				
4. Distal View				
5. Incisal/ Occlusal View				

Instructor Evaluation Rating = $\dfrac{\text{Points received}}{\text{Points possible}}$ = _____ = _____ %

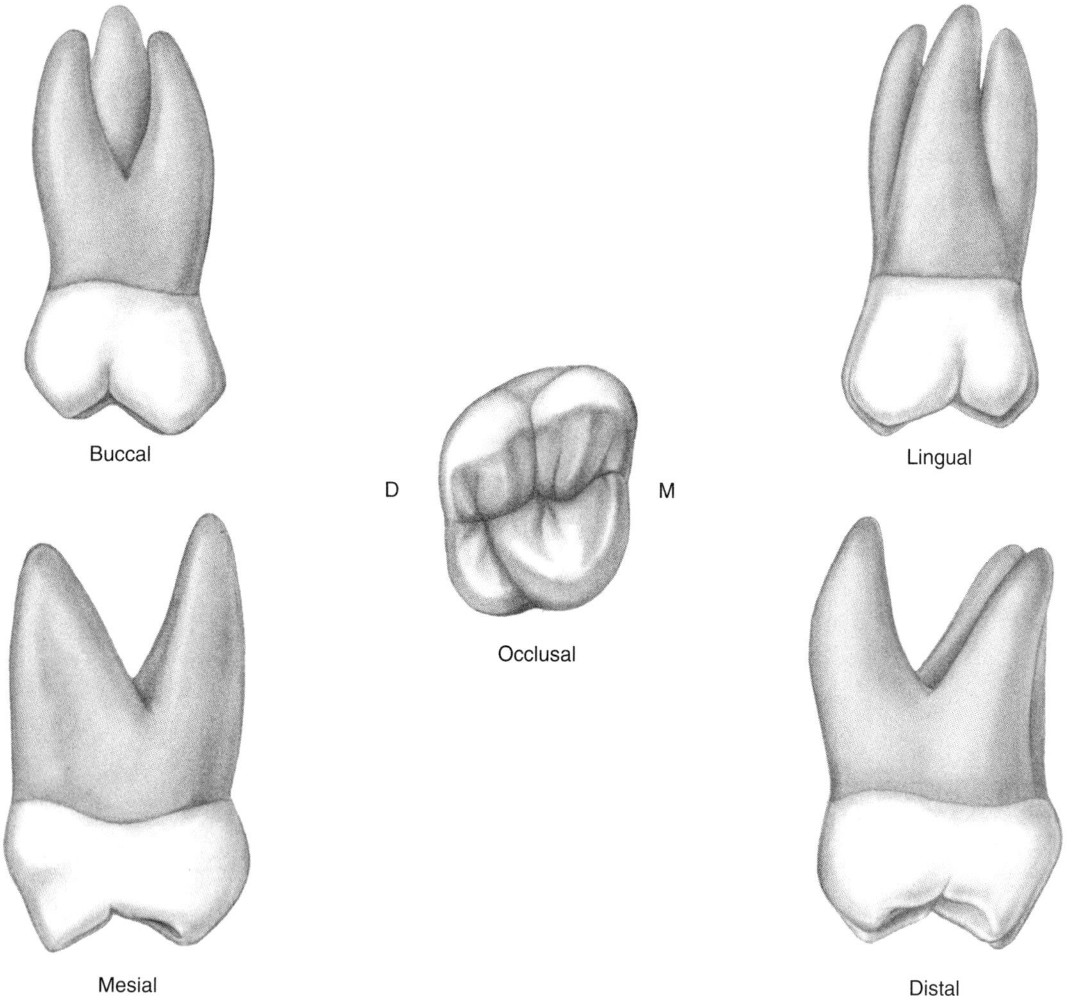

Buccal

D   M

Lingual

Occlusal

Mesial

Distal

Views of a Permanent Maxillary Right Second Molar (Rhomboidal Crown Outline)

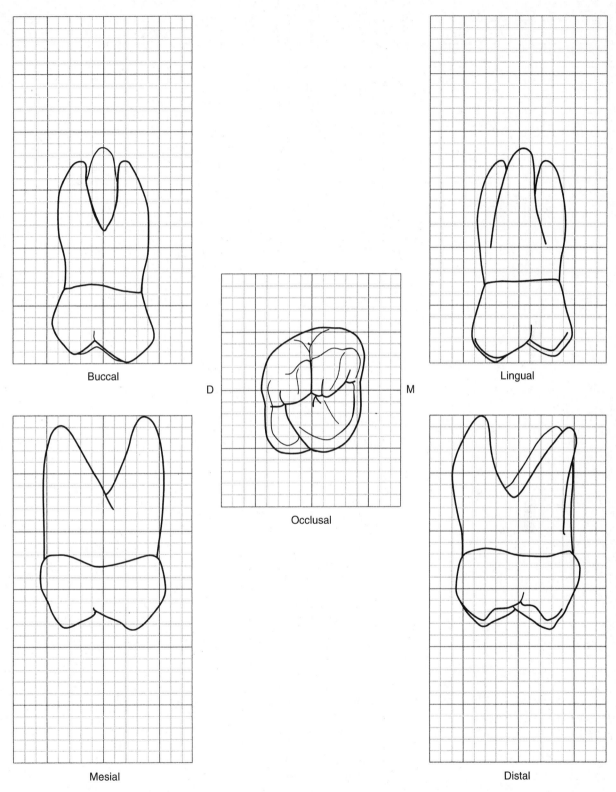

Buccal

Lingual

D   M

Occlusal

Mesial

Distal

Outline Views of a Permanent Maxillary Right Second Molar (Rhomboidal Crown Outline)

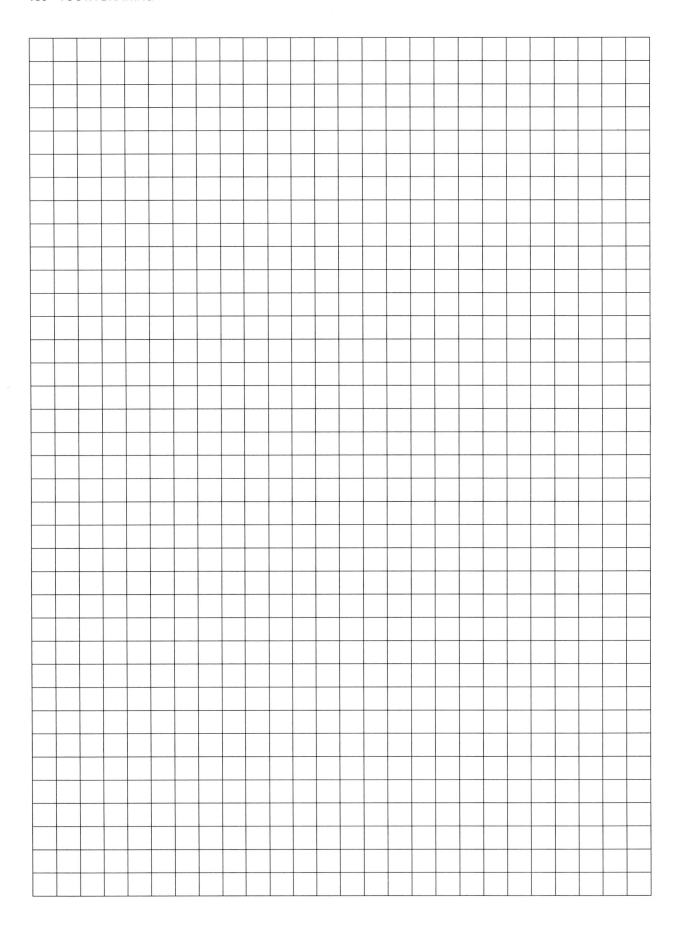

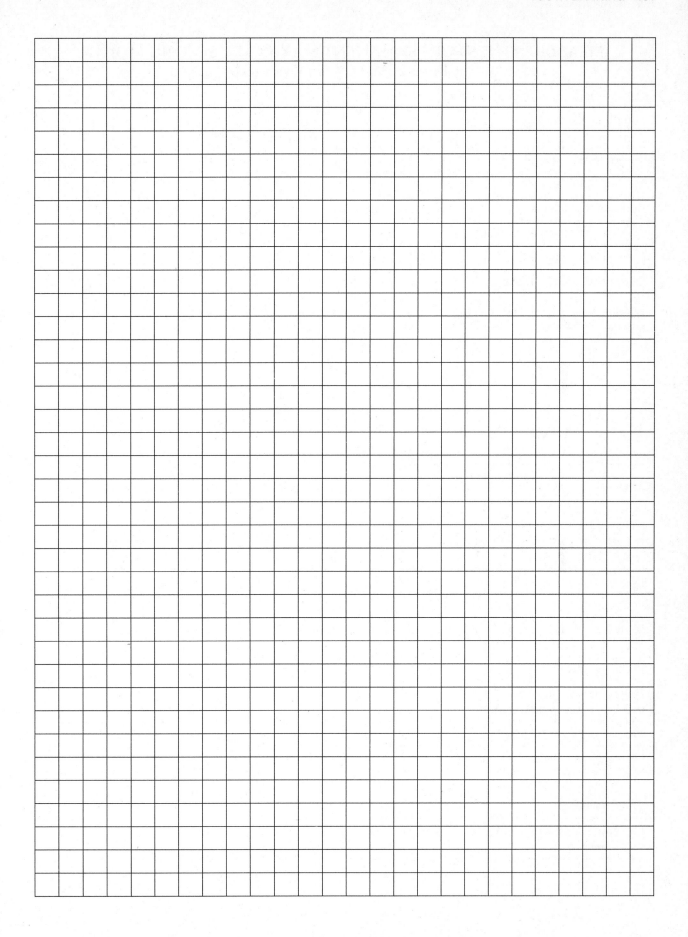

MEASUREMENTS FOR PERMANENT MAXILLARY SECOND MOLAR
(Rhomboidal Crown Outline)*

Cervico-occlusal Length of Crown	7.0
Length of Root	Buccal: 11 Lingual: 12
Mesiodistal Diameter of Crown	9.0
Mesiodistal Diameter of CEJ	7.0
Buccolingual Diameter	11.0
Buccolingual Diameter of CEJ	10.0
Curvature of CEJ—Mesial	1.0
Curvature of CEJ—Distal	0.0

*In millimeters; adapted from Nelson SJ: *Wheeler's Dental Anatomy, Physiology, and Occlusions*, ed 9, WB Saunders, Philadelphia, 2009.

CHECKLIST FOR PERMANENT MAXILLARY SECOND MOLAR
(Rhomboidal Crown Outline)

Features Noted	Features Present
Crown Features	
Occlusal table with marginal ridges and cusps with tips, ridges, inclined planes, and grooves, fossae, pits	
Less prominent oblique ridge	
Four cusps	
Mesiobuccal cusp longer than distobuccal cusp and distolingual cusp smaller	
Buccal cervical ridge	
Height of contour for the buccal is in cervical third and lingual in middle third	
Mesial contact at middle third	
Distal contact at middle third	
Root Features	
Three roots	
Furcations, root trunks, root concavities, and less divergent roots	

Name _____   Tooth Number/Name _____

Date _____   Instructor Rating _____

DRAWING EVALUATION CHECKLIST

RATING SCALE

Completely Correct = 2 points   Major Error = 0 points

Minor Error = 1 point   Note: NA (non-appropriate)

SELF-EVALUATION RATING

Five Views	Clearly Drawn	Accurate Sizing	General Features Included	Specific Features Included
1. Facial View				
2. Lingual View				
3. Mesial View				
4. Distal View				
5. Incisal/ Occlusal View				

Self-Evaluation Rating $= \dfrac{\text{Points received}}{\text{Points possible}} =$ _____ $=$ _____ %

INSTRUCTOR EVALUATION RATING

Five Views	Clearly Drawn	Accurate Sizing	General Features Included	Specific Features Included
1. Facial View				
2. Lingual View				
3. Mesial View				
4. Distal View				
5. Incisal/ Occlusal View				

Instructor Evaluation Rating $= \dfrac{\text{Points received}}{\text{Points possible}} =$ _____ $=$ _____ %

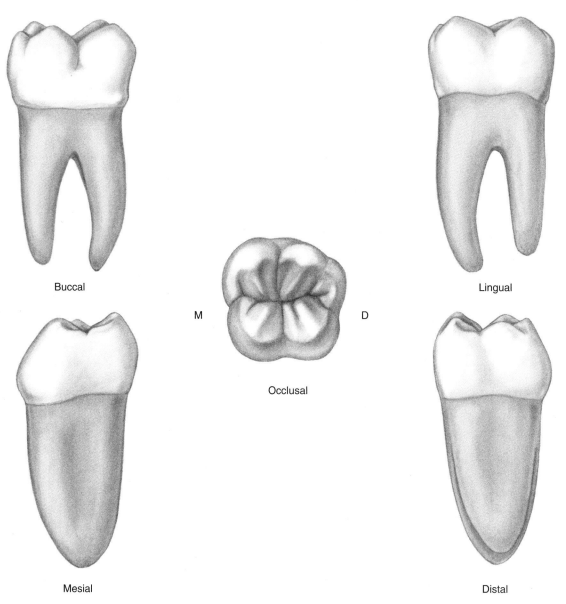

Buccal

Lingual

M   D

Occlusal

Mesial

Distal

Views of a Permanent Mandibular Right First Molar

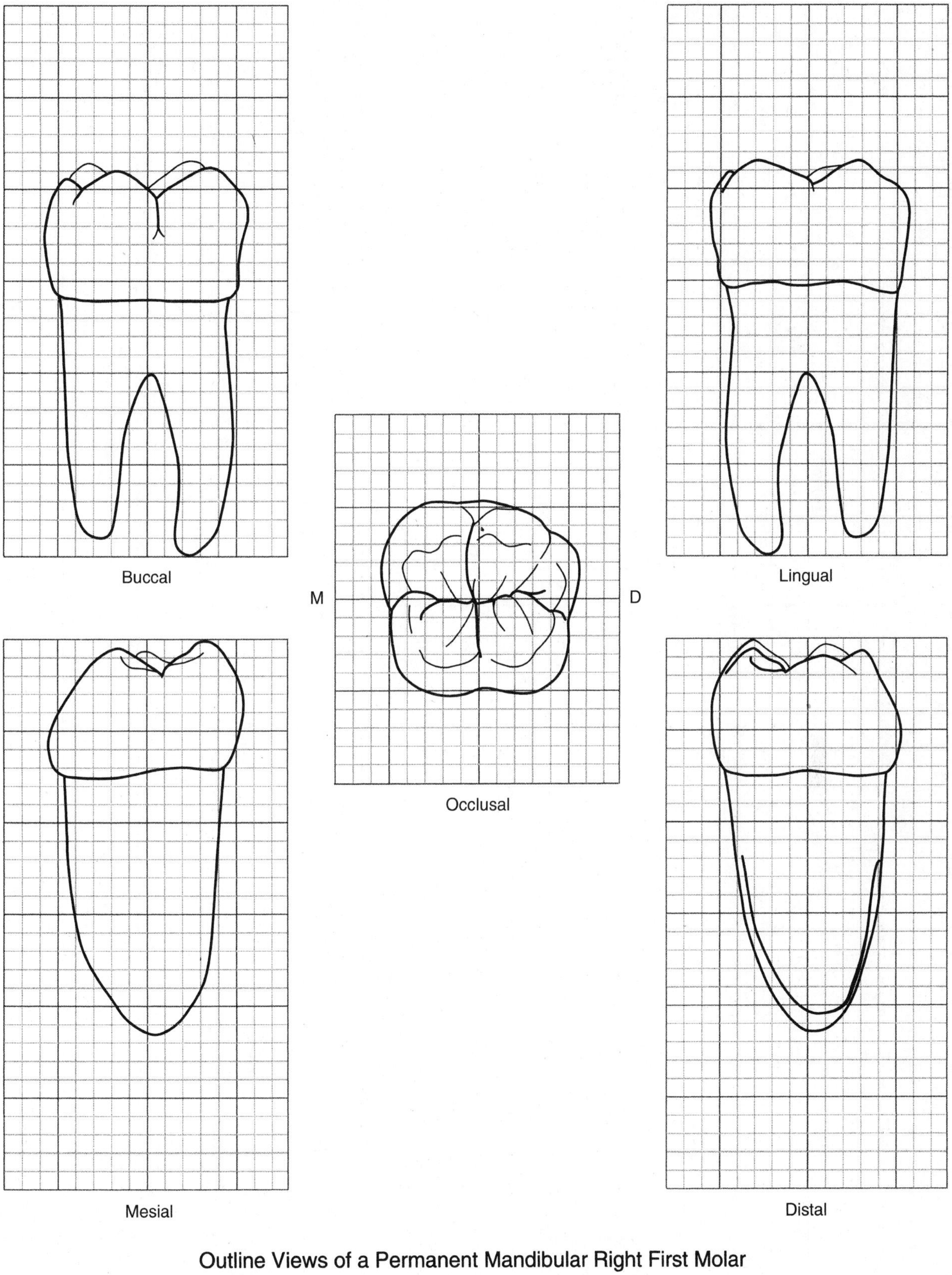

Buccal

Lingual

M   D

Occlusal

Mesial

Distal

Outline Views of a Permanent Mandibular Right First Molar

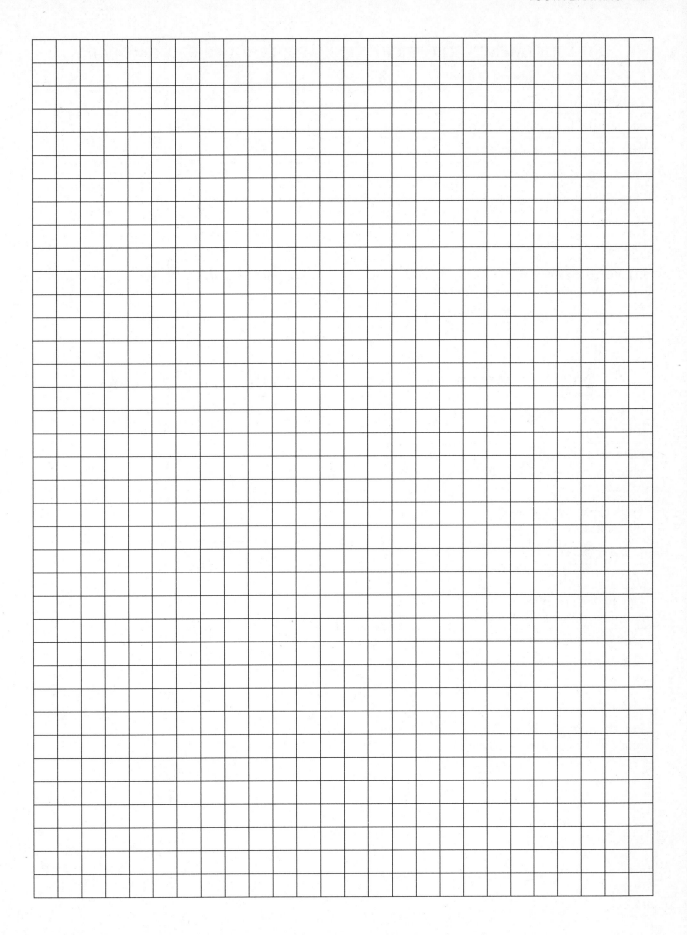

MEASUREMENTS FOR PERMANENT MANDIBULAR FIRST MOLAR*	
Cervico-occlusal Length of Crown	7.5
Length of Root	14.0
Mesiodistal Diameter of Crown	11.0
Mesiodistal Diameter of CEJ	9.0
Buccolingual Diameter	10.5
Buccolingual Diameter of CEJ	9.0
Curvature of CEJ—Mesial	1.0
Curvature of CEJ—Distal	0.0

*In millimeters; adapted from Nelson SJ: *Wheeler's Dental Anatomy, Physiology, and Occlusions*, ed 9, WB Saunders, Philadelphia, 2009.

CHECKLIST FOR PERMANENT MANDIBULAR FIRST MOLAR	
Features Noted	**Features Present**
Crown Features	
Occlusal table with marginal ridges and cusps with tips, ridges, inclined planes, and grooves, fossae, pits	
Five cusps with Y-shaped groove pattern and buccal groove	
Distal cusp is smallest with a sharp cusp	
Buccal cervical ridge	
Height of contour for the buccal is in cervical third and lingual in middle third	
Mesial and distal contact is at junction of occlusal and middle thirds	
Root Features	
Two roots	
Furcations well removed from the CEJ, root trunks, root concavities, and divergent roots	

Name _____   Tooth Number/Name _____
Date _____   Instructor Rating _____

DRAWING EVALUATION CHECKLIST

RATING SCALE
Completely Correct = 2 points   Major Error = 0 points
Minor Error = 1 point   Note: NA (non-appropriate)

SELF-EVALUATION RATING

Five Views	Clearly Drawn	Accurate Sizing	General Features Included	Specific Features Included
1. Facial View				
2. Lingual View				
3. Mesial View				
4. Distal View				
5. Incisal/ Occlusal View				

Self-Evaluation Rating = $\dfrac{\text{Points received}}{\text{Points possible}}$ = _____ = _____ %

INSTRUCTOR EVALUATION RATING

Five Views	Clearly Drawn	Accurate Sizing	General Features Included	Specific Features Included
1. Facial View				
2. Lingual View				
3. Mesial View				
4. Distal View				
5. Incisal/ Occlusal View				

Instructor Evaluation Rating = $\dfrac{\text{Points received}}{\text{Points possible}}$ = _____ = _____ %

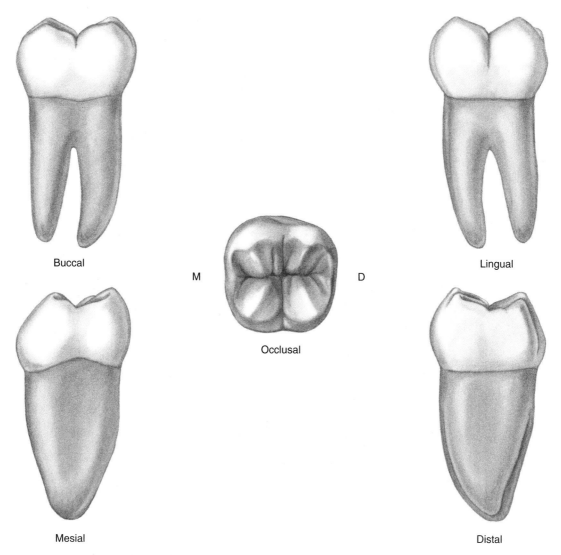

Buccal

Lingual

M   D

Occlusal

Mesial

Distal

Views of a Permanent Mandibular Right Second Molar

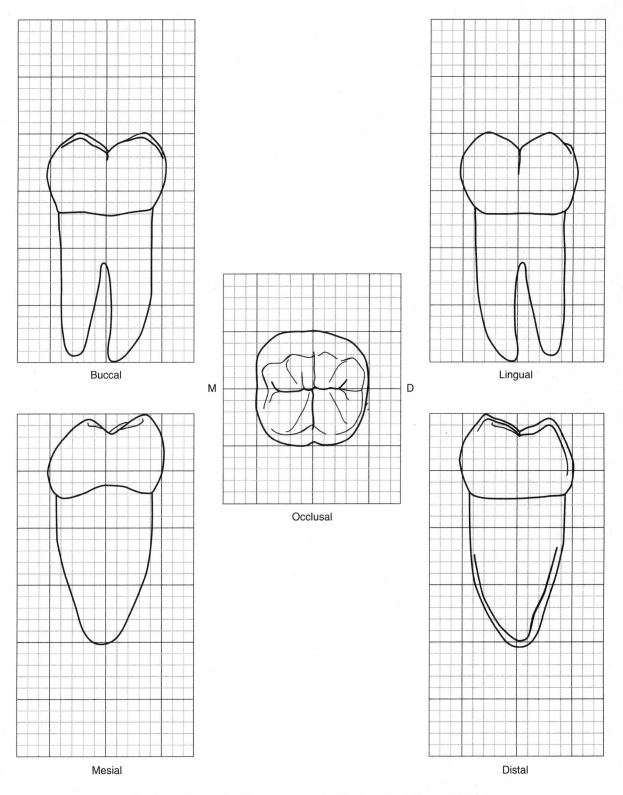

Buccal

Lingual

M   D

Occlusal

Mesial

Distal

Outline Views of a Permanent Mandibular Right Second Molar

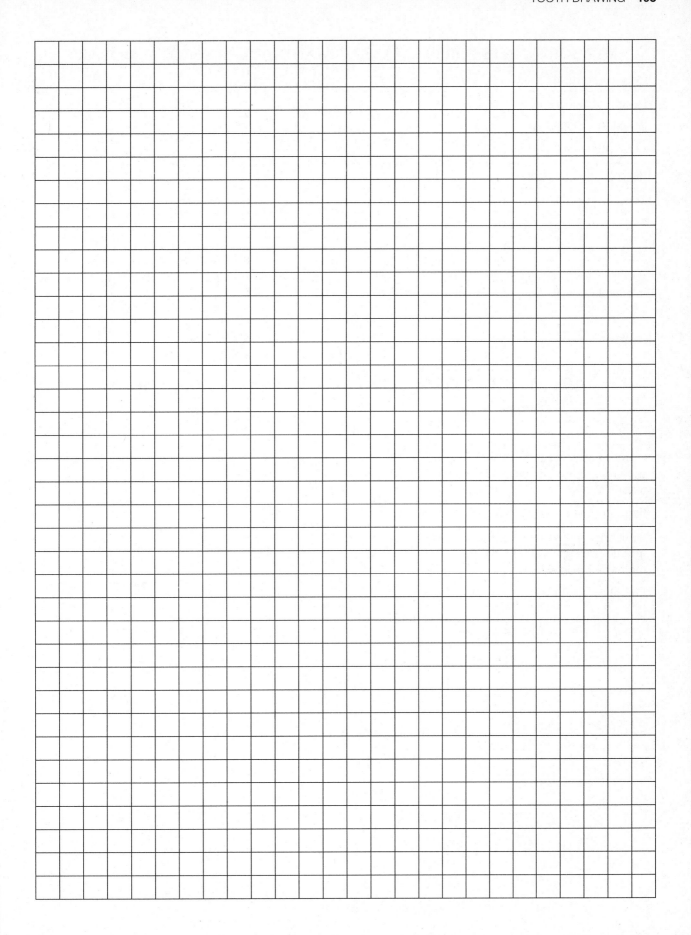

MEASUREMENTS FOR PERMANENT MANDIBULAR SECOND MOLAR*	
Cervico-occlusal Length of Crown	7.0
Length of Root	13.0
Mesiodistal Diameter of Crown	10.5
Mesiodistal Diameter of CEJ	8.0
Buccolingual Diameter	10.0
Buccolingual Diameter of CEJ	9.0
Curvature of CEJ—Mesial	1.0
Curvature of CEJ—Distal	0.0

*In millimeters; adapted from Nelson SJ: *Wheeler's Dental Anatomy, Physiology, and Occlusions*, ed 9, WB Saunders, Philadelphia, 2009.

CHECKLIST FOR PERMANENT MANDIBULAR SECOND MOLAR	
Features Noted	**Features Present**
Crown Features	
Occlusal table with marginal ridges and cusps with tips, ridges, inclined planes, and grooves, fossae, pits	
Four cusps with cross-shaped groove pattern	
Difference in height of contour for buccal and lingual from each proximal surface and wider on the mesial than distal	
Buccal cervical ridge	
Height of contour for the buccal is in cervical third and lingual in middle third	
Mesial and distal contact is at middle third	
Root Features	
Two roots	
Furcations closer to CEJ, root trunks, root concavities, and less divergent roots	

Name _____   Tooth Number/Name _____
Date _____   Instructor Rating _____

DRAWING EVALUATION CHECKLIST

RATING SCALE
Completely Correct = 2 points   Major Error = 0 points
Minor Error = 1 point   Note: NA (non-appropriate)

SELF-EVALUATION RATING

Five Views	Clearly Drawn	Accurate Sizing	General Features Included	Specific Features Included
1. Facial View				
2. Lingual View				
3. Mesial View				
4. Distal View				
5. Incisal/ Occlusal View				

$$\text{Self-Evaluation Rating} = \frac{\text{Points received}}{\text{Points possible}} = \underline{\hspace{3cm}} = \underline{\hspace{3cm}} \%$$

INSTRUCTOR EVALUATION RATING

Five Views	Clearly Drawn	Accurate Sizing	General Features Included	Specific Features Included
1. Facial View				
2. Lingual View				
3. Mesial View				
4. Distal View				
5. Incisal/ Occlusal View				

$$\text{Instructor Evaluation Rating} = \frac{\text{Points received}}{\text{Points possible}} = \underline{\hspace{3cm}} = \underline{\hspace{3cm}} \%$$

General Recommendations

When studying dental anatomy, examining extracted teeth is a valuable supplement to studying the "ideal" form noted in plastic or plaster teeth. Extracted teeth provide a more realistic concept of the anatomy of the tooth, because they have more clearly formed cusps, ridges, fossae, and pits. Variations of the ideal tooth form can also be viewed. Extracted teeth can also provide the opportunity to view relatively rare dental anomalies as well as more common ones. However, infection control should be of concern with extracted teeth in the student dental professional laboratory setting. Thus, persons who collect and inspect extracted teeth should adhere to the infection control procedures as outlined by the Occupational Safety and Health Administration (OSHA) Bloodborne Pathogens Standard as well as considerations presented by more recent research (see Selected References and Additional Resources at the end of these recommendations).

OSHA classifies extracted teeth as clinical specimens because they contain blood and, as such, contain potentially infectious material. Thus persons who collect, transport, or manipulate extracted teeth should handle them with the same precautions as specimens for biopsy. In addition, extracted teeth may include amalgam restorations, so possible pollutants when working with these teeth should be taken into consideration. Mercury vaporization and exposure is a known health hazard (see later discussion).

If not used for student study or research purposes, extracted teeth should be placed in medical waste containers unless they are returned to the patient and thus are not subject to the OSHA provisions. However, any extracted teeth containing amalgam should not be placed in medical waste containers that use incineration for final disposal, as sharps containers routinely do (see later discussion of metal recycling). If keeping the extracted tooth because the dental laboratory wants it for shade or size comparison, the disposal method followed can be the same as that outlined later when used for student study purposes.

Alternatively, more recent research has shown that extracted teeth kept for research purposes can be soaked in a solution of 10% formalin for two weeks. Tooth immersion in the formalin solution has been found effective in disinfecting both the internal and external structures of the teeth without any structure changes or pollution concerns if amalgam is present, but it will still be necessary to use standard precautions when handling the teeth. However, formalin itself is a hazardous material identified as a potential carcinogen and thus should not be used to routinely disinfect extracted teeth for student study purposes. When using formalin, the manufacturer material safety data sheet (MSDS) should be reviewed for occupational safety and health concerns and to ensure compliance with OSHA recommendations. Continued research is needed to determine the best method for treating extracted teeth before their use in research.

If kept for student study purposes, OSHA recommends that the "extracted teeth be subject to the containerization and labelling provisions of the bloodborne standard." The associated Centers for Disease Control and Prevention (CDC) guidelines state that extracted teeth should initially be collected in a "securely sealed specimen container" such as a well-constructed, wide-mouthed jar with a secure lid to prevent leakage during transport.

During the collection, the extracted teeth should be placed in a 10% solution of sodium hypochlorite (common household bleach diluted 1:10 with tap water), which then can be safely heat-sterilized. Later the contents of the jars can then be stored in a 0.2% thymol solution. At all times, the jars must be clearly marked with a biohazard symbol as well as the MSDS symbols for sodium hypochlorite and thymol. When using sodium hypochlorite and thymol, the MSDS should be reviewed for occupational safety and health concerns.

It is important to remember that, because of the risk of mercury contamination during tooth preparation, extracted teeth with amalgam cannot be saved since they cannot be safely sterilized for viewing for student study. State and local regulations should be consulted regarding the disposal of amalgam; many metal recycling companies will accept extracted teeth with amalgam. Contact a recycler and ask about company policies and about any further handling instructions needed.

In contrast with formalin preparation for research, this method of using bleach and sterilization for infection control does change the structure of the extracted teeth, but it does not prevent the use of the teeth for general student study purposes. In addition, although extracted teeth can be effectively sterilized, the CDC guidelines state that standard precautions must still be followed at all times (e.g., wearing appropriate personal protective equipment) in handling these materials by student dental professionals, because preclinical educational exercises simulate future clinical experiences.

Currently, there is no specific government-sanctioned protocol for the infection control of extracted teeth to be used for student study purposes. However, effective methods for the infection control of extracted teeth have been determined and found to be acceptable in a student dental professional laboratory setting. A recent initial study found that immersing the teeth for 48 hours in either 3% hydrogen peroxide or vinegar is equally effective as those methods previously discussed; more in-depth study needs to be completed of these less toxic and easily obtained preparations for controlling infection from extracted teeth for student study purposes. If this continues to prove to be true, the method noted below can be adapted using either of these preparations instead of bleach and sterilization.

Method for Extracted Tooth Preparation for Student Study Purposes

Step 1. Use appropriate personal protective equipment as outlined within the standard infection control precautions during preparation of the extracted teeth. Open the collection jars and pour the used bleach solution into the local access to the sewer, replacing the older solution with a new 10% bleach solution. The new solution should be left standing, surrounding the collected teeth in the jar, for at least 30 minutes.

Step 2. Using cotton pliers, place collected teeth on several layers of paper towels on a tray to protect work surfaces. Pour the newer bleach solution into the local access to the sewer, and discard collection jars and lids in any trash receptacle.

Step 3. Separate the teeth using cotton pliers, and place any teeth to be discarded, such as those with amalgam restorations, into a closed, labeled wide-mouthed jar with new 10% bleach solution, and proceed to dispose of properly (see earlier discussion).

Step 4. Place the remaining teeth to be stored into a clear zipper-lock plastic bag with a new 10% bleach solution. Place the closed bag in an ultrasonic machine for 30 minutes. Pour solution from the bag down the local access to the sewer.

Step 5. Teeth should then be covered with a wet paper towel to maintain moisture. Place teeth in plastic autoclave bags, and tape them closed. Heat-sterilize the teeth in an autoclave machine for 40 minutes at the proper temperature and pressure. Discard work materials in the biohazard waste receptacle, and wash hands. Spray tray with germicidal detergent, and allow to fully dry.

Step 6. Place the sterilized teeth into clear wide-mouthed jars, so that teeth can be viewed in storage after filling with 0.2% thymol solution before closing. Label jars according to OSHA standards with a biohazard symbol and MSDS symbols for thymol. Store the teeth under the solution at all times, so that they will not dry out and crack.

Step 7. As teeth are needed for examination, they can be removed from the jars with cotton pliers using the appropriate personal protective equipment and rinsed with tap water, soaked in a container of tap water, and rinsed again.

Selected References and Additional Resources

ADA Council on Scientific Affairs: Mercury Hygiene guidelines, *J Am Dent Assoc* 134:1498-1499, 2003.

Attam K, Talwar S, Yadav S, Miglani S: Comparative analysis of the effect of autoclaving and 10% formalin storage on extracted teeth: a microleakage evaluation, *J Conserv Dent* 12:26-30, 2009.

Batchu H, Chou H, Rakowski D, Fan PL: The effect of disinfectants and line cleaners on the release of mercury from amalgam, *J Am Dent Assoc* 137:1419-1425, 2006.

Chandki R, Mar Ru, Gunwal M, et al.: A comparison of different methods for disinfection or sterilization of extracted human teeth to be used for dental education purposes, *World J Dent* 4(1):29-31, 2013.

Dominici JT, Eleazer PD, Clark SJ, Staat RH, Scheetz JP: Disinfection/sterilization of extracted teeth for dental student use, *J Dent Educ* 65:1278-1280, 2001.

Guidelines for Infection Control in Dental Health-Care Settings, 2003, *MMWR Morb Mortal Wkly Rep* 52(RR-17):1-61, 2003.

Hashemipour MA, Mozafarinia R, Mirzadeh A, et al.: Knowledge, attitudes, and performance of dental students in relation to sterilization/disinfection methods of extracted human teeth, *Dent Res J* 10(4): 482-488, 2013.

Kumar M, Sequeira PS, Peter S, Bhat GK: Sterilization of extracted human teeth for educational use, *Indian J Med Microbiol* 23(4):256-258, 2005.

Lee JJ, Nettey-Marbell A, Cook A, Pimenta LA, Leonard R, Ritter AV: The effect of storage medium and sterilization on dentin bond strengths, *J Am Dent Assoc* 138:1599-1603, 2007.

Lolayekar NV, Bhat SV, S Bhat S: Disinfection methods of extracted human teeth, *Oral Health Comm Dent* (2):27-29, 2007.

Office of Air Quality Planning and Standards, Office of Research and Development: Mercury Study Report to Congress. Vol. II: An inventory of anthropogenic mercury emissions in the United States. Washington, DC: U.S. Environmental Protection Agency, Publication No. EPA-452/R-97-004, ES-6, 1997.

Tijare MJ, et al.: Vinegar as a disinfectant of extracted human teeth for dental educational use, *Oral Maxillofac Pathol* 18(1):14-8, 2014.

U.S. Department of Labor, Occupational Safety and Health Administration: 29 CFR Part 1910.1030. Occupational exposure to bloodborne pathogens; needlestick and other sharps injuries; final rule, *Federal Register* 66:5317-5325, 2001. Updated from and including 29 CFR Part 1910.1030. Occupational exposure to bloodborne pathogens; final rule, *Federal Register* 56:64003-64182, 1991.

U.S. Department of Labor, Occupational Safety and Health Administration: Enforcement procedures for the occupational exposure to bloodborne pathogens. Washington, DC: U.S. Department of Labor, Occupational Safety and Health Administration. Directive No. CPL 02–02–069, 2001.

UNIT I: OROFACIAL STRUCTURES

Matching

Match each item below with its best short description; each single item can only be matched once.

a.	Lymph nodes	k.	Body	u.	Buccal fat pad
b.	Exostoses	l.	Parathyroid glands	v.	Alae
c.	Periodontal ligament	m.	Vermilion zone	w.	Maxillary sinus
d.	Vestibules	n.	Mandibular symphysis	x.	Temporomandibular joint
e.	Labial frenum	o.	Fordyce spots	y.	Maxillary tuberosity
f.	Enamel	p.	Mandibular notch	z.	Linea alba
g.	External nose	q.	Anterior teeth		
h.	Parotid papilla	r.	Vertical dimension		
i.	Philtrum	s.	Buccal		
j.	Rami	t.	Tori		

1. Need to be recorded in patient's chart if palpable _____

2. Main feature of the nasal region on the face _____

3. Terminates in a thicker area of the midline of the upper lip at the tubercle of the upper lip _____

4. Mandibular bony feature between coronoid process and the condyle _____

5. Division of face into thirds from the forehead to the chin _____

6. Glands that can be palpated close to or within thyroid gland _____

7. Marking midline of mandible of the lower face _____

8. Plural of ramus that is a mandibular bony feature _____

9. Upper and lower horseshoe-shaped spaces in the oral cavity _____

10. Loss of this lip surface feature with excessive solar damage _____

11. Structure orientation that is closest to inner cheek _____

12. Oral feature at midline between the labial mucosa and alveolar mucosa on both dental arches _____

13. Elevation of tissue on inner part of buccal mucosa opposite the permanent maxillary second molar _____

14. Small yellow elevations within the oral mucosa that increase with age _____

15. Heavy horizontal part of maxilla or mandible inferior to roots of the teeth _____

16. Attaches a tooth to bony surface of alveoli _____

17. Hard outer layer of the crown of the tooth _____

18. Incisors and canines as a group within both dentitions _____

19. Slow-growing masses in premolar area noted on radiographs _____

20. Maxillary arch bony growths that may be related to occlusal trauma _____

21. Acts as a protective cushion during mastication _____

22. White ridge of hyperkeratinization extending horizontally where teeth occlude _____

23. Tissue-covered bony elevation just distal to last tooth of the maxillary arch _____

24. Nares bounded laterally by winglike cartilaginous structures _____

25. Structure inferior to the zygomatic arch and just anterior to the external ear _____

26. Structure contained within the body of maxilla _____

True or False

Assign the statement below as either true or false.

1. To palpate the lower jaw moving at the temporomandibular joint on a patient, a finger is placed on top of the temporal bone on each side during movement. _____

2. On the midline of the upper lip extending downward from the nasal septum is a vertical groove, the philtrum. _____

3. The bone underlying the mental region is the mandible, or lower jaw. _____

4. At the sides of the neck is the hyoid bone, which is suspended in the neck. _____

5. Inferior to the hyoid bone is the thyroid cartilage, which is the prominence of the larynx. _____

6. The thyroid gland, an endocrine gland, can be palpated on a patient within the midline cervical area. _____

7. The upper and lower lips meet at each corner of the mouth at the labial commissure. _____

8. The bony support for the cheek is the temporomandibular joint. _____

9. The nares are separated by the midline nasal septum. _____

10. The eyeball and all its supporting structures are contained in the orbit of the skull. _____

11. The zygomatic arch extends from just below the lateral margin of the eye toward the middle part of the external nose. _____

12. Those lingual structures closest to the palate are palatal. _____

13. Deep within each vestibule is the vestibular fornix, where the pink labial mucosa or buccal mucosa meets the alveolar mucosa. _____

14. An excess amount of linea alba on either the buccal mucosa or tongue can be associated with certain oral parafunctional habits. _____

15. The maxilla is a single bone with a movable articulation with the temporal bones at each temporomandibular joint. _____

16. The vertically placed canine eminence is especially prominent on each side of the maxilla. _____

17. The dense pad of tissue located just distal to the last tooth of the mandibular arch is the retromolar pad. _____

18. The permanent maxillary anterior teeth are supplied by the anterior superior alveolar artery, with the permanent maxillary posterior teeth supplied by the posterior superior alveolar artery. _____

19. All of the permanent mandibular teeth are supplied by branches of the anterior superior alveolar artery. _____

20. The alveolar process is the bony extension for both the maxilla and mandible that contain each alveolus. _____

21. The inner parts of the lips are lined by a pink buccal mucosa. _____

22. Both the labial and buccal mucosa may vary in coloration, as do other regions of the oral mucosa, in individuals with pigmented skin. _____

23. The interdental gingiva is the gingival tissue between adjacent teeth adjoining attached gingiva. _____

24. The inner surface of the gingival tissue where each tooth faces a space is the gingival sulcus. _____

25. The inside of the mouth is known as the oral cavity proper. _____

26. Posteriorly, the opening from the oral cavity proper into the pharynx is the palate. _____

27. The palatine tonsils are located on the lateral side of the tongue. _____

28. A midline ridge of tissue on the hard palate is the retromolar pad. _____

29. The palatine rugae are firm, irregular ridges of tissue radiating from the incisive papilla and median palatine raphe. _____

30. The sulcus terminalis separates the base from the body of the tongue. _____

Ordering

Place the following items in the correct order as indicated.

1. In what order should these facial surface features be placed, going from superior to inferior on the face?

    _____ a. Infraorbital region

    _____ b. Mental region

    _____ c. Orbital region

    _____ d. Frontal region

2. In what order should these oral region features be placed, going from the outer part to inner part of the upper lip?

    _____ a. Vermilion zone

    _____ b. Mucocutaneous junction

    _____ c. Tubercle of the upper lip

    _____ d. Philtrum

3. In what order should these facial surface features be placed, going from medial to lateral on the face?

    _____ a. Nasal region

    _____ b. External ear

    _____ c. Infraorbital region

    _____ d. Zygomatic region

4. In what order should these facial surface features be placed, going from superior to inferior on the face?

    _____ a. Philtrum

    _____ b. Root of the nose

    _____ c. Nares

    _____ d. Apex of the nose

5. In what order should these neck surface features be placed, going from superior to inferior on the neck?

    _____ a. Thyroid cartilage

    _____ b. Hyoid bone

    _____ c. Mandible

    _____ d. Thyroid gland

6. In what order should these facial surface features be placed, going from medial to lateral on the face?

_____ a. Mandibular condyle

_____ b. Labial commissures

_____ c. Mandibular notch

_____ d. Coronoid process

7. In what order should these oral cavity features be placed, going from superior to inferior on the maxillary arch?

_____ a. Attached gingiva

_____ b. Marginal gingiva

_____ c. Mucogingival junction

_____ d. Alveolar mucosa

8. In what order should these oral cavity features be placed, going from anterior to posterior on the palate?

_____ a. Palatal rugae

_____ b. Incisive papilla

_____ c. Maxillary incisors

_____ d. Attached gingiva

9. In what order should these oral cavity features be placed, going from anterior to posterior on the dorsal surface of the tongue?

_____ a. Body of the tongue

_____ b. Apex of the tongue

_____ c. Base of the tongue

_____ d. Sulcus terminalis

10. In what order should these features of both the larynx and pharynx be placed, going from superior to inferior within the neck area?

_____ a. Nasopharynx

_____ b. Larynx

_____ c. Oropharynx

_____ d. Laryngopharynx

UNIT II: DENTAL EMBRYOLOGY

Matching

Match each item with the best short description below; each single item can only be matched once.

a.	Cloacal membrane	k.	Mesoderm	u.	Meckel cartilage
b.	Differentiation	l.	Morphogenesis	v.	Secondary palate
c.	Ectoderm	m.	Neural crest cells	w.	Cap stage
d.	Embryonic period	n.	Neuroectoderm	x.	Primary palate
e.	Endoderm	o.	Oropharyngeal membrane	y.	Supernumerary teeth
f.	Fetal period	p.	Placenta	z.	Frontonasal process
g.	Fusion	q.	Preimplantation period		
h.	Induction	r.	Primitive streak		
i.	Maturation	s.	Proliferation		
j.	Mesenchyme	t.	Somites		

1. Period when fertilization and implantation occur _____

2. Period involving the embryo growing into fetus _____

3. Second week to eighth week of prenatal development _____

4. Action of one group of cells on another that leads to the establishment of the developmental pathway in the responding tissue _____

5. Controlled cellular growth and accumulation of byproducts _____

6. Change in identical embryonic cells to become distinct, both structurally and functionally _____

7. Development of specific tissue structure or differing form due to embryonic cell migration and inductive interactions _____

8. Attainment of adult function and size due to proliferation, differentiation, and morphogenesis _____

9. Originates directly from the epiblast layer _____

10. Future dermis, muscle, bone of the body _____

11. Layer of cuboidal cells within the embryo _____

12. Considered by many histologists to be fourth embryonic layer _____

13. Prenatal organ that joins pregnant woman and developing embryo _____

14. Furrowed, rod-shaped thickening in the middle of embryonic disc _____

15. Differentiates to form most of the connective tissue of the head _____

16. Location of future primitive mouth of embryo _____

17. Location of future terminal end of embryo's digestive tract _____

18. Specialized group of cells that differentiates from the ectoderm _____

19. Elimination of groove between two adjacent swellings of tissue or processes on embryo surface _____

20. Mesoderm that additionally differentiates and begins to divide into paired cuboidal aggregates of cells _____

21. Most disappears as the bony mandible forms by intramembranous ossification _____

22. Forms as a bulge of tissue at most cephalic end of embryo _____

23. Initially serves as a partial separation between the developing oral cavity proper and the nasal cavity _____

24. Will give rise to posterior two-thirds of hard palate _____

25. Abnormal initiation may result in development of one or more extra teeth _____

26. Stage of unequal growth in different parts of tooth bud _____

True or False

Assign the statement below as either true or false.

1. The face and its related tissue begin to form during the sixth week of prenatal development. _____

2. All three embryonic layers are involved in facial development. _____

3. Facial development is completed for the most part during the twelfth week of prenatal development. _____

4. The overall growth of the face is in a superior and posterior direction in relationship to the cranial base. _____

5. The stomodeum initially appears as a shallow depression in the embryonic surface ectoderm at the cephalic end. _____

6. Oral epithelium is derived from ectoderm as a result of embryonic folding. _____

7. The paired maxillary processes fuse at the midline to form the mandibular arch. _____

8. The placodes are rounded areas of specialized, thickened ectoderm found at the location of developing special sense organs. _____

9. The paired medial nasal processes also fuse internally and grow inferiorly on the inside of the stomodeum, forming the intermaxillary segment. _____

10. The upper lip is formed when each maxillary process fuses with each nearby medial nasal process. _____

11. The beginnings of the embryo's hollow tube are derived from the anterior part of the midgut. _____

12. The stacked bilateral outer swellings of tissue that appear inferior to the stomodeum and include the mandibular arch are the branchial pouches. _____

13. Palatal fusion allows the fusion of swellings or tissue from different surfaces of the embryo. _____

14. The intermaxillary segment gives rise to the secondary palate. _____

15. The secondary palate will give rise to the anterior third of the hard palate. _____

16. In the future, the neural crest cells will become involved in the formation of components of the nervous system, melanocyte pigment cells. _____

17. The tongue develops during the fourth to eighth weeks of prenatal development. _____

18. Tongue development begins as a triangular median swelling, the tuberculum impar. _____

19. The copula is formed from the fusion of mesenchyme of mainly the third and parts of the fourth branchial arches. _____

20. The foramen cecum is the beginning of the thymus. _____

21. The oral epithelium grows deeper into the ectomesenchyme and is induced to produce a layer called the dental membrane. _____

22. A depression results in the deepest part of each tooth bud of dental lamina and forms the enamel knot. _____

23. The dental papilla will produce the future dentin and pulp for the inner part of the tooth. _____

24. Three embryologic structures, the enamel organ, dental papilla, and dental sac, are considered together to be the tooth germ. _____

25. After the inner enamel epithelium differentiates into preameloblasts, the outer cells of the dental papilla are induced by the preameloblasts to differentiate into ameloblasts. _____

26. Developmental disturbances can occur within each stage of odontogenesis, affecting the physiologic processes taking place. _____

27. The initial teeth for both dentitions develop in the anterior maxillary region. _____

28. The primary dentition develops during only the embryonic period of prenatal development. _____

29. The second stage of odontogenesis is considered bud stage and occurs at the beginning of the eighth week of prenatal development for the primary dentition. _____

30. The dental sac will produce the periodontium, the supporting tissue types of the tooth. _____

Ordering

Place the following items in the correct order as indicated.

1. In what order should these events during prenatal development be noted, going from earlier to later in time span?

    _____ a. Conception

    _____ b. Preimplantation period

    _____ c. Fetal period

    _____ d. Embryonic period

2. In what order should these events occurring during prenatal development be noted, going from earlier to later in time span?

    _____ a. Mitosis

    _____ b. Implantation

    _____ c. Meiosis

    _____ d. Sperm and egg union

3. In what order should these structures present during prenatal development be noted, going from earlier to later in time span?

    _____ a. Fetus

    _____ b. Embryo

    _____ c. Blastocyst

    _____ d. Zygote

4. In what order should these prenatal structures be placed, going from closest to farthest in relationship to the endometrium lining the uterus?

    _____ a. Amniotic cavity

    _____ b. Hypoblast layer

    _____ c. Epiblast layer

    _____ d. Yolk sac

5. In what order should these prenatal structures be placed, going from superior to inferior in relationship to the embryo?

_____ a. Midgut

_____ b. Hindgut

_____ c. Foregut

_____ d. Oropharyngeal membrane

6. In what order should these structures present during prenatal development be noted, going from earlier to later in time span?

_____ a. Stomodeum

_____ b. Mandibular processes

_____ c. Mandibular arch

_____ d. Primitive mouth

7. In what order should these prenatal structures be placed, going from superior to inferior in relationship to the embryo?

_____ a. Hyoid arch

_____ b. Third branchial arch

_____ c. Mandibular arch

_____ d. Fourth branchial arch

8. In what order should these prenatal structures be placed, going from superior to inferior in relationship to the embryo?

_____ a. Frontonasal process

_____ b. Maxillary processes

_____ c. Mandibular arch

_____ d. Stomodeum

9. In what order should these structures present during palatal development be noted, going from earlier to later in time span?

_____ a. Primary palate

_____ b. Intermaxillary segment

_____ c. Palatal shelves

_____ d. Secondary palate

10. In what order should these structures present during tongue development be noted, going from earlier to later in time span?

_____ a. Copula

_____ b. Lateral lingual swellings

_____ c. Epiglottic swelling

_____ d. Tuberculum impar

11. In what order should these events during odontogenesis be noted, going from earlier to later in time span?

_____ a. Bud stage

_____ b. Cap stage

_____ c. Initiation stage

_____ d. Bell stage

12. In what order should these layers of the enamel organ be placed, going from the outer part to inner part in relationship to the overall tooth?

_____ a. Outer enamel epithelium

_____ b. Stellate reticulum

_____ c. Inner enamel epithelium

_____ d. Stratum intermedium

UNIT III: DENTAL HISTOLOGY

Matching

Match each item below with its best short description; each one item can only be matched once.

a.	Anaphase	k.	Mucoperiosteum	u.	Interglobular dentin
b.	Basement membrane	l.	Nucleoplasm	v.	Lamina dura
c.	Cell	m.	Organ	w.	Sulcular epithelium
d.	Connective tissue	n.	Organelles	x.	Fibroblast
e.	Cytoplasm	o.	Prophase	y.	Gingival recession
f.	Epithelium	p.	Rete ridges	z.	Attrition
g.	Granulation tissue	q.	System		
h.	Histology	r.	Telophase		
i.	Interphase	s.	Tissue		
j.	Metaphase	t.	von Ebner		

1. Study of microscopic structure and function of cells and tissue _____
2. Smallest living unit of organization within the body _____
3. Collection of similarly specialized cells that work in the body _____
4. Independent body part formed from tissue _____
5. Organs functioning together within the body _____
6. Semifluid part contained within cell membrane boundary _____
7. Chromatin condenses into chromosomes _____
8. Mitotic spindle forms during cell division _____
9. Migration of chromatids to opposite poles by mitotic spindle _____
10. Reappearance of the nuclear membrane _____

11. Cells between divisions is involved in this time period _____
12. Specialized, metabolically active structures within the cell _____
13. Fluid part within the nucleus of the cell _____
14. Tissue type that covers and lines external and internal body surfaces _____
15. Extensions of epithelium into connective tissue as appear on histologic section _____
16. Thin, acellular, chemical-based structure located between any form of epithelium and its underlying connective tissue _____
17. By weight, most abundant type of basic tissue in body _____
18. Immature connective tissue with few fibers and increased amount of blood vessels _____
19. Consisting of a mucous membrane combined with the periosteum of the adjacent bone _____

20. Glands present in the submucosa deep to the lamina propria of the circumvallate lingual papillae _____

21. Wearing away of hard tissue as a result of tooth-to-tooth contact _____

22. Can cause root dentin to be exposed with a thin layer of cementum lost _____

23. Only primary mineralization has occurred within predentin _____

24. Part of the alveolar bone proper that is present on radiographs _____

25. Most common cell in the periodontal ligament _____

26. Stands away from the tooth, creating a gingival sulcus _____

True or False

Assign the statement below as either true or false.

1. The interdental gingiva assumes a nonvisible concave form between the facial and lingual gingival surfaces called the col. _____

2. Healthy attached gingiva is pink in color, with some areas of melanin pigmentation possible. _____

3. In some cases, a free gingival groove separates the sulcular gingiva from the marginal gingiva. _____

4. The dentogingival junction is the direct junction between the tooth surface and the periodontal ligament. _____

5. The sulcular epithelium is of an orthokeratinized type, with its cells tightly packed. _____

6. Before the eruption of the tooth and after enamel maturation, the ameloblasts secrete a basal lamina on the surface that serves as a part of the primary epithelial attachment. _____

7. An endocrine gland is a gland having a duct associated with it. _____

8. Saliva also supplies the minerals for subgingival calculus formation. _____

9. Mucoserous acini have both a group of mucous cells surrounding the lumen and a serous demilune. _____

10. More than one myoepithelial cell can sometimes be found on a single acinus. _____

11. The submandibular salivary gland is the smallest, most diffuse, and only unencapsulated major salivary gland. _____

12. The parathyroid glands are visible or palpable during an extraoral examination of a patient. _____

13. Tissue fluid drains from the surrounding region into the lymphatic vessels as lymph. _____

14. Each lymphatic nodule has a germinal center, containing many immature lymphocytes. _____

15. Intraoral tonsillar tissue consists of nonencapsulated masses of lymphoid tissue located in the lamina propria of the oral mucosa. _____

16. The palatine tonsils are four rounded masses of variable size located between the anterior and posterior faucial pillars. _____

17. The lingual tonsil is an indistinct layer of diffuse lymphoid tissue located on the lateral surface of the tongue. _____

18. Each lateral wall of the nasal cavity has three projecting structures, or nasal conchae, that extend inward. _____

19. The nasal cavity is lined by a respiratory mucosa, like the rest of the respiratory system. _____

20. The moist mucus forms a deep, invasive system in the respiratory mucosa. _____

21. The underlying histologic states of its components provide a clue to the clinical features noted visibly with the periodontium, whether in a healthy or diseased state. _____

22. The mature cementum consists of mainly calcium hydroxyapatite with the chemical formula of $Ca_{10}(PO_4)_6(OH)_2$. _____

23. The trabecular bone appears less uniformly radi-opaque and more porous than the uniformly radiopaque lamina dura. _____

24. With the loss of teeth, a patient becomes edentu-lous, either partially or completely. _____

25. During the chronic advanced type of periodon-tal disease of periodontitis, the basal bone is always lost. _____

26. The epithelial rests of Malassez are present within the alveolar process but can become cystic. _____

27. The periodontal ligament is wider near the apex and cervix of the tooth. _____

28. During mastication and speech, certain forces are exerted on a tooth, such as rotational, tilting, extrusive, or intrusive. _____

29. The interradicular group of the alveolodental ligament is found only between the alveolar crests of neighboring teeth. _____

30. The dentogingival ligament is the most exten-sive of the gingival fiber group. _____

Ordering

Place the following items in the correct order as indicated.

1. In what order should these cellular structures be placed, going from outer part to inner part of the cell?

_____ a. Cell membrane

_____ b. Nucleolus

_____ c. Nucleus

_____ d. Nuclear membrane

2. In what order should these components of the body be noted, going from a simple to a more complex type of organization?

_____ a. Cell

_____ b. Organ

_____ c. Tissue

_____ d. System

3. In what order should these phases present during mitosis be noted, going from earlier to later in time span?

_____ a. Anaphase

_____ b. Prophase

_____ c. Metaphase

_____ d. Telophase

4. In what order should these bone layers be placed, going from superficial to deeper layers in the tissue?

_____ a. Compact bone

_____ b. Endosteum

_____ c. Periosteum

_____ d. Cancellous bone

5. In what order should these steps present during endochondrial ossification be noted, going from earlier to later in time span?

_____ a. Formation of primary ossification centers

_____ b. Osteoblasts penetrate cartilage

_____ c. Production of osteoid in layers

_____ d. Cartilage disintegrates

6. In what order should these components of skeletal muscle be placed, going from superficial to deeper layers in relationship to the muscle bundle?

_____ a. Myofilaments

_____ b. Myofibers

_____ c. Myofibrils

_____ d. Muscle fascicles

7. In what order should these layers of orthokera-tinized stratified squamous epithelium be placed, going from superficial to deeper layers in the tissue?

_____ a. Keratin layer

_____ b. Basal layer

_____ c. Prickle layer

_____ d. Granular layer

8. In what order should these salivary glands be noted, going from largest to smallest as related to individual size?

_____ a. von Ebner gland

_____ b. Submandibular gland

_____ c. Parotid gland

_____ d. Sublingual gland

9. In what order should these components of salivary glands be placed, going from larger to smaller in size as well as superficial to deeper within the gland?

_____ a. Lobes

_____ b. Acini

_____ c. Capsule

_____ d. Lobules

10. In what order should these components of salivary glands be placed, going from superficial near the capsule to deeper in the gland?

_____ a. Intercalated duct

_____ b. Acinus

_____ c. Striated duct

_____ d. Excretory duct

11. In what order should these components of the thyroid gland be placed, going from larger to smaller in size as well as superficial to deeper within the gland?

_____ a. Lobes

_____ b. Follicles

_____ c. Capsule

_____ d. Lobules

12. In what order should these components of a lymph node be noted, going the same way as the flow of lymph entering and exiting the node?

_____ a. Efferent vessel

_____ b. Lymphatic vessel

_____ c. Afferent vessel

_____ d. Hilus

13. In what order should these components of a lymph node be placed, going from larger to smaller in size as well as superficial to deeper within the node?

_____ a. Lymphatic nodule

_____ b. Trabeculae

_____ c. Capsule

_____ d. Germinal center

14. In what order should these events involving the ameloblasts during odontogenesis be placed, going from earlier to later in time span?

_____ a. Forming enamel matrix from Tomes process

_____ b. Actively transporting materials for mineralization

_____ c. Becoming part of reduced enamel epithelium

_____ d. Removing water and organic material from enamel

15. In what order should these zones in pulp be placed, going from the outer pulpal wall near the dentin to the inner part of the pulp?

_____ a. Pulpal core

_____ b. Cell-rich zone

_____ c. Cell-free zone

_____ d. Odontoblastic layer

16. In what order should these fiber groups of the alveolodental ligament of the periodontal ligament be placed, going from the cementoenamel junction to the tooth apex?

_____ a. Horizontal group

_____ b. Oblique group

_____ c. Alveolar crest group

_____ d. Apical group

UNIT IV: DENTAL ANATOMY

Matching

Match each item below with its best short description; each one item can only be matched once.

a.	Anatomic root	k.	Furcation	u.	Occlusal table
b.	Bicuspid	l.	Mamelons	v.	Transverse ridge
c.	Bifurcated	m.	Occlusion	w.	Trifurcated
d.	Bruxism	n.	Overjet	x.	Curve of Wilson
e.	Centric relationship	o.	Palmer Notation Method	y.	Wisdom
f.	Cervical ridge	p.	Primate spaces	z.	Articular fossa
g.	Cingulum	q.	Sextant		
h.	Contact	r.	Adult teeth		
i.	Cuspids	s.	Supplemental grooves		
j.	Diastema	t.	Supporting cusps		

1. Other name for the permanent dentition that is commonly used _____

2. Tooth numbering system commonly used during orthodontic therapy _____

3. Used to describe anatomic alignment of teeth and their relationship to rest of masticatory system _____

4. Division of each dental arch into three parts based on relationship to the midline _____

5. Part of root covered by a layer of cementum _____

6. Raised, rounded area on the cervical third of lingual surface of anterior teeth _____

7. Rounded enamel extensions on the incisal ridge from either labial or lingual views _____

8. Mainly viewed as the open contact between permanent maxillary central incisors _____

9. Older term for the canines that is still used today _____

10. Occlusal surface is bordered by marginal ridges to create inner surface _____

11. Joining of two triangular ridges crossing occlusal surface from labial to lingual outline _____

12. Secondary grooves on the occlusal surface that appear as shallow, more irregular linear depressions _____

13. Older term for the premolar that is still used today _____

14. Maxillary first premolars having two root branches _____

15. Common name for the third molar teeth _____

16. Area between two or more of the root branches before division from root trunk _____

17. Maxillary molars with three root branches _____

18. Spaces between primary maxillary lateral incisor and canine and between the primary mandibular canine and first molar _____

19. Ridge more prominent on primary molars than any similar structure on permanent molar _____

20. Cause of extensive wear of incisal edge of primary incisor _____

21. End point of closure of the mandible _____

22. Maxillary dental arch naturally overhanging mandibular arch facially _____

23. Area on the proximal surfaces of teeth with the same-arch neighbors _____

24. Concave curve that results when a frontal section is taken through each set of both maxillary and mandibular molars _____

25. Cusps that function during centric occlusion _____

26. Depression on inferior aspect of temporal bone _____

True or False

Assign the statement below as either true or false.

1. The anteroposterior curvature is called the curve of Wilson, which is produced by the curved alignment of all the teeth and is especially evident when viewing the posterior teeth from the buccal. _____

2. Phase three of arch development begins when the canines wedge themselves between the lateral incisors and the first premolars. _____

3. Open contacts allow for areas of food impaction from opposing cusps, called plunging cusps, resulting in trauma to the interdental gingiva. _____

4. Overbite is measured in millimeters with the tip of a periodontal probe. _____

5. If a tooth is lost for a longer period, the neighboring teeth usually become more upright in an effort to fill the edentulous space. _____

6. Triangular grooves separate a marginal ridge from the triangular ridge of a cusp and at their terminations form the triangular fossae. _____

7. The contact area of each of the posterior teeth is wider than anterior teeth, is usually located to the lingual of center, and is nearer the same level on each proximal surface. _____

8. Some inclined planes are functional and thus involved in the occlusion of the teeth. _____

9. The crown of each posterior tooth has an occlusal surface as its masticatory surface, bordered by the raised marginal ridges, which are located on both the facial surface and lingual surface. _____

10. Most permanent maxillary first premolars are trifurcated, having two root branches in the apical third, with a buccal root and a lingual root. _____

11. Permanent maxillary second premolars erupt between 10 and 12 years of age. _____

12. There is one form of permanent mandibular second premolars, the tricuspidate form, which is a three-cusp type. _____

13. The permanent dentition is also sometimes considered the nonsuccedaneous dentition, because all of these permanent teeth succeed primary predecessors. _____

14. The molars, because of their tapered shape and their prominent cusp, function to pierce or tear food during mastication. _____

15. A tooth numbering system that is commonly used in orthodontic therapy is the Palmer Notation Method. _____

16. The joint capsule outer layer is a synovial membrane, which consists of a thin connective tissue with nerves and blood vessels. _____

17. The central area of the temporomandibular joint disc is vascularized and has innervation. _____

18. Lateral deviation of the mandible, or lateral excursion, which involves shifting the lower jaw to one side, occurs during mastication. _____

19. Not all patients with temporomandibular disorders have abnormalities in the joint disc or even in the joint itself; most symptoms seem to originate from the muscles. _____

20. The Palmer Notation Method is also known as the *Military Tooth Numbering System.* _____

21. The permanent dentition period begins with the eruption of the primary mandibular central incisors. _____

22. The mixed dentition period occurs between approximately 6 and 12 years of age. _____

23. A growth center is located in the head of each mandibular condyle before an individual reaches maturity. _____

24. Lateral deviation involves only gliding movements of contralateral temporomandibular joints in their respective joint cavities. _____

25. When the teeth of the occlusion are in the position of centric occlusion, each tooth of one arch is in occlusion with two others in the opposing arch, except for a few teeth. _____

26. Premature contacts are where one or two teeth contact after the other teeth. _____

27. The permanent canine should usually be the only tooth in function during lateral occlusion. _____

28. The permanent central incisors are closest to the midline, and the permanent lateral incisors are the second teeth from the midline. _____

29. The pulp chamber of the permanent maxillary central incisor has two sharp elongations: the mesial and distal pulp horns. _____

30. The lingual surface of the crown of a permanent maxillary lateral incisor is narrower than the labial surface. _____

31. The crown of a permanent mandibular central incisor is quite asymmetrical from the labial view. _____

32. Because of their tapered shape and prominent cusp, the permanent canines function to pierce or tear food during mastication. _____

33. The mesial half of the crown of a permanent maxillary canine resembles a part of a premolar, and the distal half resembles a part of a permanent incisor. _____

34. Like anterior teeth, multirooted permanent premolars and molars originate as a single root on the base of the crown. _____

35. Since the permanent maxillary first molar has a buccal and lingual root, it also has two furcations. _____

36. The lingual cusp is slightly displaced to the distal, which helps to distinguish the permanent maxillary right second premolar from the left. _____

37. Both types of permanent mandibular premolars can present difficulties during instrumentation due to narrow lingual surfaces combined with the lingual inclination of the crown. _____

38. The permanent mandibular first molar has the most complex developmental groove pattern of all the permanent mandibular molars. _____

39. The two roots of a permanent mandibular first molar are smaller, shorter, and less divergent than those of a second molar. _____

40. The pulp cavity of a permanent mandibular first molar is more likely to have three root canals—distal, mesiobuccal, and mesiolingual—and five pulp horns. _____

41. Permanent maxillary third molars, along with the mandibular third molars, commonly exhibit partial anodontia and thus are congenitally missing. _____

42. The defining oblique ridge is less prominent on the permanent maxillary second molar than on the first molar. _____

43. From the mesial, the mesial contact area of a permanent maxillary second molar is larger, and the cervical flattening or concavity is never as pronounced as in a first molar. _____

44. The two roots on permanent maxillary second molars are smaller than the first molars. _____

45. Loss of the tooth is followed by mesial inclination and drift of the maxillary second molar into the open arch space, and the mandibular first molar, if present, also supererupts. _____

46. On the permanent maxillary first molar, the two marginal ridges and two cusp ridges of the four major cusps are found bordering the occlusal table on the buccal and lingual margins. _____

47. The crown of any primary tooth is short in relation to its total length. _____

48. Overall, the dentin of the primary dentition is thicker than that of the permanent counterparts. _____

49. From the labial aspect, the crown of the primary maxillary central incisor appears wider mesiodistally than incisocervically, the opposite of its permanent successor. _____

50. The crown of the primary maxillary first molar does not resemble any other crown of either dentition. _____

Ordering

Place the following items in the correct order as indicated.

1. In what order should the following general dental terms be placed, going from the largest number of teeth included in an adult to the smallest number of teeth?

   _____ a. Dentition

   _____ b. Quadrant

   _____ c. Arch

   _____ d. Sextant

2. In what order should the following line angles of an anterior tooth be placed, going from mesial to distal for the front of the tooth and then in the same direction for the back of the tooth?

   _____ a. Mesiolabial

   _____ b. Distolabial

   _____ c. Mesiolingual

   _____ d. Distolingual

3. In what order should the following permanent incisors be placed, going from largest in overall size to smallest?

   _____ a. Mandibular lateral

   _____ b. Mandibular central

   _____ c. Maxillary central

   _____ d. Maxillary lateral

4. In what order should be following permanent teeth be placed according to their approximate eruption dates, going from earlier to later in time span?

   _____ a. Mandibular central incisors

   _____ b. Maxillary canines

   _____ c. Maxillary first premolars

   _____ d. Mandibular first molars

5. In what order should the following cusps of the permanent mandibular first molar be placed, going from largest in overall size to smallest?

   _____ a. Mesiolingual

   _____ b. Distolingual

   _____ c. Distobuccal

   _____ d. Mesiobuccal

6. In what order should the following cusps of the permanent maxillary first molar be placed, going from largest in overall size to smallest?

   _____ a. Mesiolingual

   _____ b. Distolingual

   _____ c. Distobuccal

   _____ d. Mesiobuccal

7. In what order should the following events during formation of the primary dentition be placed, going from earlier to later in time span?

_____ a. All teeth have started mineralization

_____ b. Beginning of tooth mineralization

_____ c. Completion of full dentition

_____ d. Eruption of first tooth into oral cavity

8. In what order should these skull features be placed, going from anterior to posterior on the skull?

_____ a. Postglenoid process

_____ b. Articular eminence

_____ c. Zygomatic arch

_____ d. Articular fossa

9. In what order should the following permanent premolars be placed, going from largest in overall size to smallest?

_____ a. Mandibular first

_____ b. Mandibular second

_____ c. Maxillary first

_____ d. Maxillary second

10. In what order should be following permanent teeth be placed according to their approximate eruption dates, going from earlier to later in time span?

_____ a. Maxillary lateral incisors

_____ b. Mandibular canines

_____ c. Maxillary second premolars

_____ d. Mandibular second molars

UNIT II: DENTAL EMBRYOLOGY CASE STUDY 1

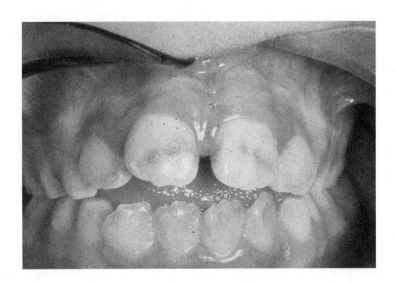

Age	23 years	**Scenario**
Sex	☐ Male ☒ Female	The patient visits the dentist regularly every 6 months, but this is a new dental office since she has moved recently and to a region without water fluoridation. She has begun having difficulty with homecare on her small-sized teeth. She also regularly chews sugared gum. She says she has always had staining on her teeth. Her previous dentist recommended full-coverage crowns but said that she needed to wait until her teeth were fully erupted. She also used to suck her thumb when she was a child. When younger, she briefly lived in an area with naturally higher levels of fluoride in the drinking water. Clinical photograph of her dentition was taken.
Height	5 feet, 8 inches	
Weight	120 pounds	
BP	85/65 mm Hg	
Chief Complaint	*"Can we whiten my front teeth as soon as possible?"*	
Medical History	None	
Current Medications	Birth control pills	
Social History	First-grade teacher	

* Courtesy of Margaret J. Fehrenbach, RDH, MS.

1. What dental disturbance is present in her anterior teeth of both arches?
   A. Concrescence
   B. Enamel dysplasia
   C. Dentinal dysplasia
   D. Chronic pulpitis

2. Which of the following cell types were MAINLY disturbed so as to cause her chief concern?
   A. Odontoblasts
   B. Fibroblasts
   C. Ameloblasts
   D. Cementoblasts

3. During which of the following stage(s) of odontogenesis does this dental disturbance of the anterior teeth occur?
   A. Bud stage
   B. Initiation stage
   C. Cap or bell stages
   D. Apposition and maturation stages

4. What is the EXACT type of staining present in this patient?
   A. Extrinsic
   B. Intrinsic
   C. Transient
   D. Temporary

5. Because the patient has an unusual bite noted with her occlusion, what is also present on the masticatory surface of her mandibular anterior teeth?
   A. Attrition
   B. Perikymata
   C. Mamelons
   D. Occlusal tables

UNIT II: DENTAL EMBRYOLOGY CASE STUDY 2

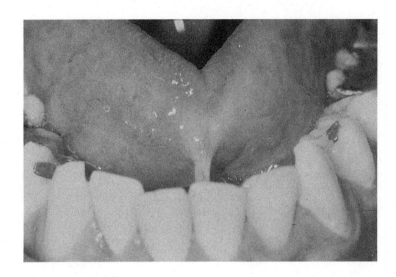

Age	52 years	Scenario
Sex	☒ Male ☐ Female	The new patient has had a moderate speech impediment since childhood but has never had speech lessons, orofacial myofunctional therapy, or any surgical procedures, even though they were all suggested to his parents. Mandibular anteriors show crowding and moderate amounts of supragingival calculus on the lingual surface. A clinical photograph of his mandibular anterior sextant was taken.
Height	5 feet, 10 inches	
Weight	224 pounds	
BP	115/82 mm Hg	
Chief Complaint	*"My teeth on the lower jaw are getting more crowded."*	
Medical History	Repaired right kneecap	
Current Medications	None	
Social History	Historian at local university	

1. What orofacial disturbance is present in this patient?
   A. Gemination
   B. Fusion
   C. Ankyloglossia
   D. Cleft uvula

2. The orofacial disturbance MAINLY involves what part of the oral cavity?
   A. Lingual frenum
   B. Lingual gingiva
   C. Soft palate
   D. Soft tissue of tongue

3. In what week of prenatal development does the associated orofacial structure involved in the dental disturbance begin its specific development?
   A. First week
   B. Second week
   C. Third week
   D. Fourth week

4. Which of the following is the superficial demarcation of fusion noted in the associated structure(s) involved in the orofacial disturbance?
   A. Lateral lingual swellings
   B. Copula
   C. Epiglottic swelling
   D. Tuberculum impar

5. During what prenatal developmental time does the associated structure involved in the orofacial disturbance complete its fusion?
   A. Fetal period
   B. Embryonic period
   C. Initiation stage
   D. Maturation stage

UNIT II: DENTAL EMBRYOLOGY CASE STUDY 3

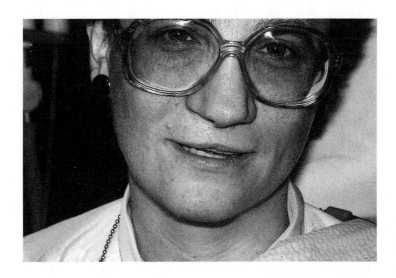

		Scenario
Age	45 years	The new patient had surgery as a young child on the right part of her upper lip from a birth defect. Had speech lessons as child but is still embarrassed by her slight speech impediment as well as the slight scar remaining. No defects noted in her oral cavity. She has moderate inflammation of the maxillary arch and does admit to mouth breathing. Moderate amounts of supragingival calculus also noted throughout with slight to moderate xerostomia and hyposalivation. A file photograph for the patient record was taken.
Sex	☐ Male ☒ Female	
Height	5 feet, 3 inches	
Weight	105 pounds	
BP	105/68 mm Hg	
Chief Complaint	*"Why do I have so much tartar on my teeth?"*	
Medical History	Premenopausal and allergy to pollens; past smoker	
Current Medications	Decongestants and short-term hormone replacement therapy	
Social History	Mother of six children	

1. Which of the following developmental disturbances has affected this patient?
   A. Fusion
   B. Cleft palate
   C. Cleft lip
   D. Spina bifida

2. Which of the following processes is MAINLY involved in the patient's developmental disturbance?
   A. Maxillary process
   B. Lateral nasal process
   C. Mandibular process
   D. Frontonasal process

3. This developmental disturbance in the patient occurs MORE commonly and MORE severely in which of the following populations?
   A. Men
   B. Women
   C. Adolescent
   D. Geriatric

4. Which of the following statements is CORRECT concerning this patient's developmental disturbance?
   A. Only hereditary etiologic factors noted
   B. May be associated with other abnormalities
   C. Only occurs unilaterally
   D. Occurs mainly on the right side

5. During which prenatal developmental time does this developmental disturbance in the patient occur?
   A. Pre-implantation period
   B. Embryonic period
   C. Initiation stage
   D. Apposition stage

UNIT II: DENTAL EMBRYOLOGY CASE STUDY 4

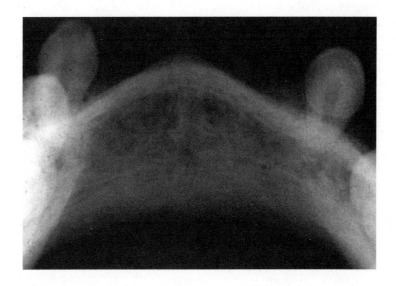

Age	23 years	**Scenario**
Sex	☒ Male ☐ Female	The new patient is being seen at a community dental clinic after referral by the school nurse. He appears older than he is because his hair is sparse. He is unable to tolerate a warm environment and needs special measures to keep a normal body temperature since birth. He is saving to have dental implants placed through a reduced-fee program at the local dental school. An occlusal radiograph was taken of his mandibular anterior sextant along with other radiographs.
Height	6 feet, 3 inches	
Weight	165 pounds	
BP	112/84 mm Hg	
Chief Complaint	*"I need to know if I can have those implant teeth put in and when it can occur."*	
Medical History	Hearing difficulty due to genetic defect	
Current Medications	None	
Social History	Aspiring actor after finishing high school drama with honors	

1. Which of the following developmental disturbances is present with this patient?
   A. Fetal alcohol syndrome
   B. Down syndrome
   C. Ectodermal dysplasia
   D. Spina bifida

2. Which of the following can be noted in these developmental disturbance cases?
   A. Various levels of intellectual disability
   B. Indistinct philtrum and thin upper lip
   C. Abnormalities of skin, hair, nails
   D. Epicanthic folds around eyes

3. The noted developmental disturbance has involvement with which of the following etiologic factors?
   A. Teratogenic
   B. Hereditary
   C. Radiation
   D. Drug usage

4. What of the following can be used to help this patient and would serve in both a cosmetic and a functional purpose for the present time?
   A. Wheelchair
   B. Dentures
   C. Surgical removal
   D. Speech therapy

5. The structures involved with this developmental disturbance are formed during which prenatal developmental time?
   A. Fetal period
   B. Embryonic period
   C. Initiation stage
   D. Maturation stage

UNIT II: DENTAL EMBRYOLOGY CASE STUDY 5

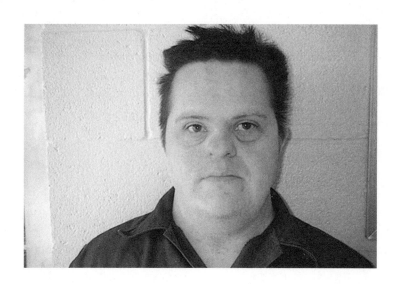

Age	26 years	**Scenario**
Sex	☒ Male ☐ Female	The patient is attending his welcome appointment but has further appointments set up with his new dental office, as he does with his regular speech therapist. A patient photograph was taken for his file. He has microdontia and malformed teeth in an oral cavity that has an undersized bone structure. The roots of his teeth are small and conical, and he mouth breathes. He has moderate early bone loss with chronic periodontal disease and xerostomia. Needs to have a complete examination and a full mouth series of radiographs taken, as well as appointments for his oral care.
Height	5 feet, 4 inches	
Weight	245 pounds	
BP	110/85 mm Hg	
Chief Complaint	*"I need my teeth cleaned."*	
Medical History	Sleep apnea and hypothyroidism related to genetic disturbance	
Current Medications	Thyroid hormone and antiseizure medication	
Social History	Lives at group home after being home schooled and works part time at a library	

1. Which of the following developmental disturbances is present with this patient?
    A. Fetal alcohol syndrome
    B. Down syndrome
    C. Ectodermal dysplasia
    D. Spina bifida

2. During what prenatal developmental event does this disturbance occur?
    A. Meiosis
    B. Mitosis
    C. Maturation stage
    D. Mesoderm formation

3. What was MAINLY involved during this developmental disturbance?
    A. Ectopic pregnancy
    B. Infective teratogen
    C. Trisomy 21
    D. Neural tube defect

4. Which of the following may be present with this patient?
    A. Fissures of the tongue
    B. Enlarged tongue
    C. Hyperplasia of lingual papillae
    D. Furrowed upper lip

5. Which of the following is the CORRECT number of chromosomes present after the joining of the sperm and ovum but may not have occurred for this patient?
    A. 12
    B. 23
    C. 46
    D. 92

UNIT III: DENTAL HISTOLOGY CASE STUDY 1

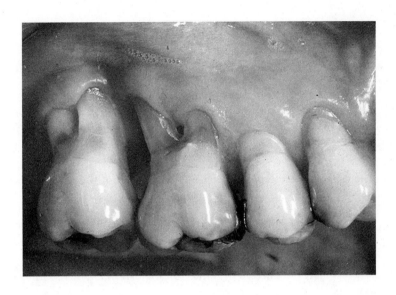

Age	57 years	Scenario
Sex	☐ Male ☒ Female	The new patient regularly visited the dentist until her dentist retired 15 years ago. She has been diagnosed with chronic periodontal disease (periodontitis). Clinical photographs were taken of the facial view of each quadrant, along with a full mouth series of of radiographs. Exposed roots were noted throughout, with moderate to severe bone loss. Slight bleeding and moderate mobility were also observed throughout. She notes that her teeth are slightly loose.
Height	5 feet, 11 inches	
Weight	190 pounds	
BP	102/78 mm Hg	
Chief Complaint	*"Why do my teeth look so long lately?"*	
Medical History	Past history of skin cancer	
Current Medications	None	
Social History	Retired tennis player	

1. What part of the alveolar process has the patient lost between the roots of her molars?
   A. Basal bone
   B. Alveolar crest bone
   C. Interdental septum
   D. Interradicular septum

2. What fiber group of the periodontal ligament is the FIRST group to be affected by periodontal disease in this patient?
   A. Alveolar crest group
   B. Horizontal group
   C. Oblique group
   D. Apical group

3. Both the patient's lost alveolar process and altered periodontal ligament are considered part of which of the following orofacial structures?
   A. Periodontium
   B. Alveolodental ligament
   C. Principal fiber groups
   D. Temporomandibular joint

4. What part of each of the posterior teeth was FIRST lost as a result of the root exposure?
   A. Predentin
   B. Secondary dentin
   C. Cellular cementum
   D. Coronal enamel

5. Which cell population has been MOST active in removing the alveolar process in the patient because of the chronic periodontal disease?
   A. Ameloblast
   B. Osteoclast
   C. Odontoblast
   D. Odontoclast

UNIT III: DENTAL HISTOLOGY CASE STUDY 2

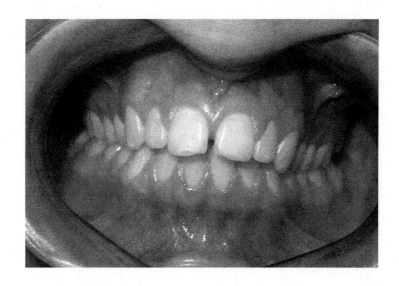

Age	32 years	**Scenario**	
Sex	☒ Male ☐ Female	The patient has not been to the dentist in 5 years and is new to the office. His previous dentist told him that he needed to brush more. A clinical facial photograph was taken of his dentition, along with a full mouth series of radiographs. Moderate bleeding is noted, but no bone loss was noted on radiographs. He does not regularly brush or floss his teeth and does not routinely take his medication or test his blood since the housing market crashed locally in the last year.	
Height	5 feet, 11 inches		
Weight	280 pounds		
BP	110/85 mmHg		
Chief Complaint	*"Why do my teeth keep bleeding when I floss?"*		
Medical History	Type II diabetes mellitus		
Current Medications	Oral diabetes medication		
Social History	Real estate agent with four children		

1. What type of mucosa is involved in the inflammation noted in the patient?
   A. Lining mucosa
   B. Specialized mucosa
   C. Masticatory mucosa
   D. Paranasal mucosa

2. Which fiber group associated with the periodontal ligament is the FIRST group to be affected with inflammation in this patient?
   A. Gingival fiber group
   B. Alveolar crest group
   C. Horizontal group
   D. Oblique group

3. What is the MAIN underlying cause of this patient's gingival bleeding when flossing?
   A. Thickening of the junctional epithelium
   B. Repair of the lamina propria's blood vessels
   C. Increased blood vessels in the lamina propria
   D. Increased collagen production around blood vessels

4. What is the EXACT term used when dealing with the patient's present periodontal condition?
   A. Active gingivitis
   B. Chronic gingivitis
   C. Active periodontitis
   D. Chronic periodontitis

5. What is the patient's histologic situation that is present in BOTH the epithelium and lamina propria at the dentogingival junction?
   A. Smooth interface at basement membrane between tissue types
   B. Decreased numbers of migrating white blood cells
   C. Formation of rete pegs and connective tissue papillae
   D. All signs of chronic inflammation throughout tissue types

UNIT III: DENTAL HISTOLOGY
CASE STUDY 3

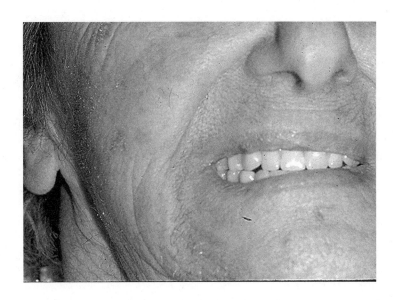

Age	82 years	Scenario
Sex	☐ Male ☒ Female	The patient is seeing the dentist for the first time after entering the extended care facility that has services available on site. She has a moderate level of dry mouth noted. Her maxillary and mandibular complete dentures do not fit comfortably. A clinical photograph was taken with both her upper and lower dentures in place and while trying to occlude.
Height	5 feet, 3 inches	
Weight	112 pounds	
BP	95/78 mm Hg	
Chief Complaint	*"Why does my mouth feel so dry?"*	
Medical History	Early stages of Alzheimer disease; used to smoke	
Current Medications	Antidepressant	
Social History	Former nurse for community public health facility	

1. What is the term used to describe her dry mouth condition?
   A. Erosion
   B. Abfraction
   C. Hyposalivation
   D. Xerostomia

2. Which is the largest salivary gland present in the patient?
   A. Parotid
   B. Submandibular
   C. Sublingual
   D. Von Ebner

3. What salivary gland usually produces the MOST saliva in the oral cavity?
   A. Parotid
   B. Submandibular
   C. Sublingual
   D. Von Ebner

4. What part of each of the jaws is still completely present in this patient?
   A. Basal bone
   B. Alveolar process
   C. Interdental septum
   D. Interradicular septum

5. The patient is experiencing diminished length of the lower third of the face; what is this termed?
   A. Increase in facial Golden Proportions
   B. Loss of vertical dimension
   C. Partially edentulous state
   D. Mesial drift and supereruption

UNIT III: DENTAL HISTOLOGY
CASE STUDY 4

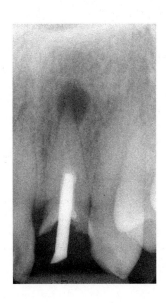

Age	45 years	Scenario
Sex	☒ Male ☐ Female	This is a patient of record. When he was in his twenties, the affected tooth was treated with endodontic therapy by a specialist because of a dental anomaly. He is now experiencing pain on percussion when chewing in the area. A periapical radiograph of the involved tooth was taken. An abscess at the apex of the tooth was noted. He has noted a bad taste in the mouth but no longer chews spit tobacco.
Height	6 feet, 4 inches	
Weight	180 pounds	
BP	100/62 mm Hg	
Chief Complaint	*"Can you fix my painful broken tooth?"*	
Medical History	Osteoarthritis in knees and past use of spit tobacco	
Current Medications	Over-the-counter herbal preparations	
Social History	High school basketball coach	

1. What is the dental anomaly that was present in this tooth?
   A. Fusion
   B. Gemination
   C. Dens in dente
   D. Peg lateral

2. Why is the patient experiencing oral pain with this tooth?
   A. Secondary dentin is filling pulp chamber
   B. Inflammatory edema is pressing on nerves
   C. Inert material is extruding from the pulp
   D. Apical bone is forming at the apex

3. Why did the tooth break in the patient's oral cavity?
   A. Darkening of the tooth
   B. Failure during lobular division
   C. Loss of tooth vitality
   D. Placement of gutta-percha

4. What is the MAIN path by which pulpal infection travels to the surrounding apical periodontium and causes an abscess?
   A. Apical foramen
   B. Pulp horns
   C. Accessory canals
   D. Dentinal tubules

5. Which of the following cell populations can produce additional pulp tissue after an injury such as the one this patient has experienced?
   A. Odontoblasts
   B. Red blood cells
   C. White blood cells
   D. Undifferentiated mesenchymal cells

UNIT III: DENTAL HISTOLOGY
CASE STUDY 5

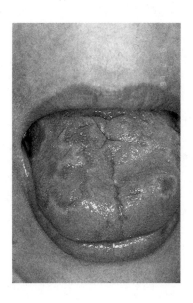

		Scenario
Age	32 years	The new patient is a recent emigrant and regularly visited her dentist in her native country. After her last visit to the dental school, she now uses an electric toothbrush. A clinical photograph of her tongue was taken. She says she has always had this condition of the dorsal surface of the tongue, along with slight soreness. She brushes her tongue regularly as directed but does not know why this keeps occurring.
Sex	☐ Male ☒ Female	
Height	5 feet, 2 inches	
Weight	120 pounds	
BP	90/78 mm Hg	
Chief Complaint	*"Why does the top of my tongue look funny?"*	
Medical History	Osteoporosis	
Current Medications	Calcium supplements	
Social History	Chef in restaurant	

1. What is the condition noted on the patient's dorsal surface of the tongue?
   A. Fissured tongue
   B. Central papillary atrophy
   C. Geographic tongue
   D. Burning mouth syndrome

2. What type of lingual papillae is MAINLY involved in this tongue condition?
   A. Filiform
   B. Fungiform
   C. Circumvallate
   D. Foliate

3. What type of oral mucosa is MAINLY associated with this condition on the dorsal surface of the tongue?
   A. Masticatory
   B. Lining
   C. Specialized
   D. Paranasal

4. Which of the following is associated with sensory neuron processes when the patient is working at her career?
   A. Taste pore
   B. Taste cells
   C. Supporting cells
   D. Surrounding tongue epithelium

5. What area of the patient's tongue has NEVER had any fungiform lingual papillae?
   A. Sulcus terminalis
   B. Apex or tip of tongue
   C. Body of the tongue
   D. Near filiform lingual papillae

UNIT IV: DENTAL ANATOMY
CASE STUDY 1

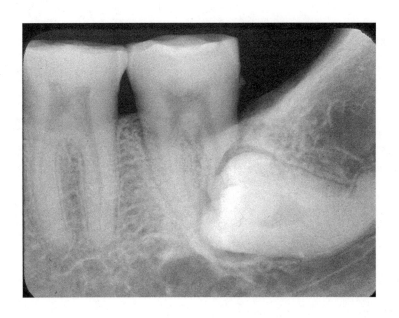

Age	25 years	Scenario
Sex	☒ Male ☐ Female	As a patient of record, he had orthodontic therapy at a specialist's office as an adolescent. He now wears a mouthguard at night because of a moderate-level bruxism and early symptoms of temporomandibular joint disorder. A periapical radiograph was taken of the most painful area of his lower jaw. No lesions in the mouth were noted. He has generalized moderate attrition, but he has been classified as having a low risk of caries.
Height	6 feet, 1 inch	
Weight	190 pounds	
BP	98/67 mm Hg	
Chief Complaint	*"Why does my lower jaw hurt even when using my mouthguard?"*	
Medical History	None	
Current Medications	None	
Social History	Professor of chemistry	

1. What is the condition noted on the patient's radiograph that is probably causing him his symptom of oral pain?
   A. Cyst formation
   B. Microdontia
   C. Partial anodontia
   D. Impacted third molar

2. Which of the following are features of the tooth that is causing the patient's discomfort?
   A. Three roots
   B. Four pulp horns
   C. Consistent crown form
   D. Square crown outline

3. When does the tooth that is causing the patient's discomfort usually complete its roots?
   A. 10 to 14 years
   B. 13 to 17 years
   C. 17 to 21 years
   D. 18 to 25 years

4. What are the opaque structures noted in the pulp chambers of some of the mandibular posterior teeth?
   A. Denticles
   B. Pulp stones
   C. Sialoliths
   D. Enamel pearls

5. Which structure is located on the patient's temporal bone anterior to the articular fossa of the temporo-mandibular joint?
   A. Joint capsule
   B. Articular eminence
   C. Synovial membrane
   D. Articulating surface of the condyle

UNIT IV: DENTAL ANATOMY
CASE STUDY 2

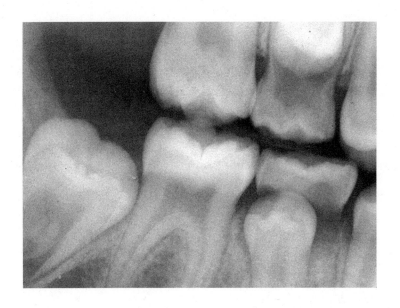

Age	11 years	Scenario
Sex	☒ Male ☐ Female	As a patient of record, he has been to the dentist once before at age 7, and enamel sealants were placed on all erupted permanent posterior teeth. A posterior bitewing radiograph was taken on both sides. Four posterior teeth are loose, and four teeth are partially erupted. Inflammation is noted around loose and partially erupted teeth.
Chief Complaint	*"Why do my back teeth feel real loose when I wiggle them?"*	
Medical History	None	
Current Medications	None	
Social History	Likes to play baseball, wants to be a firefighter	

1. On which teeth were enamel sealants probably placed at his last dental appointment?
   A. First premolars
   B. Second premolars
   C. First molars
   D. Second molars

2. Which partially erupted teeth may require placement of enamel sealants at the next appointment because of their increased risk of caries?
   A. First premolars
   B. Second premolars
   C. First molars
   D. Second molars

3. Which of the following teeth within his dentition may be loose and ready to be exfoliated?
   A. *S*
   B. *T*
   C. #2
   D. #30

4. The crown of which posterior tooth appears similar to the crown anatomy of one of the nearby loose teeth?
   A. *S*
   B. *T*
   C. #2
   D. #30

5. Which of the following teeth may have already been exfoliated?
   A. *S*
   B. *T*
   C. #2
   D. #30

UNIT IV: DENTAL ANATOMY CASE STUDY 3

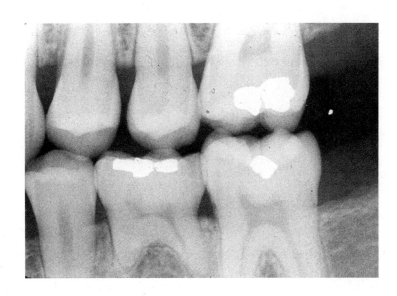

		Scenario
Age	25 years	She is a new patient. At age 6, enamel sealants were placed on four teeth that were later restored due to failure at the margins. She had four permanent posterior teeth extracted at age 13 because of extensive caries and four more at age 20 because of impaction. Her most recent dentist told her that some of her "adult" teeth were never going to erupt. Two posterior bitewing radiographs were taken. Small mandibular posterior teeth were noted bilaterally. She is having difficulty with homecare on her smaller-sized teeth. She regularly chews sugared gum and does not live in a water-fluoridated region.
Sex	☐ Male ☒ Female	
Height	5 feet, 6 inches	
Weight	180 pounds	
BP	98/75 mm Hg	
Chief Complaint	*"Why is one of my back teeth on each side smaller than the rest?"*	
Medical History	None	
Current Medications	None	
Social History	Hairdresser with three small children	

1. For which permanent posterior teeth does the patient exhibit a case of partial anodontia?
   A. Second premolars
   B. First molars
   C. Second molars
   D. Third molars

2. Which permanent posterior teeth did the patient have extracted earlier as an adolescent?
   A. Second premolars
   B. First molars
   C. Second molars
   D. Third molars

3. Which permanent posterior teeth did the patient have extracted later as a young adult?
   A. Second premolars
   B. First molars
   C. Second molars
   D. Third molars

4. Which permanent posterior teeth have been restored in the patient because of failure of the enamel sealants?
   A. Second premolars
   B. First molars
   C. Second molars
   D. Third molars

5. Of the teeth now present in the patient, which of the following mandibular teeth have two roots?
   A. Second premolars
   B. First molars
   C. Second molars
   D. Third molars

UNIT IV: DENTAL ANATOMY
CASE STUDY 4

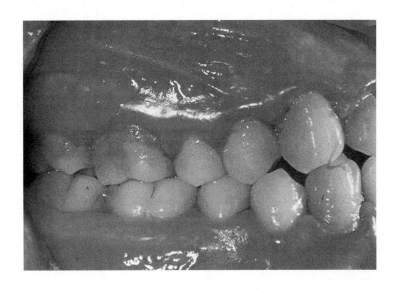

Age	42 years	Scenario
Sex	☒ Male ☐ Female	The new patient is very nervous in the dental chair. He has not visited a dentist in 12 years. He had orthodontic therapy as a teenager but did not wear a retainer as suggested. Permanent third molars were extracted at age 20. He says he grinds his teeth at night. A clinical photograph was taken of both sides, along with a full mouth series of radiographs. No caries were noted. Moderate inflammation of the gingiva is present, with deposits noted throughout. He has always used a soft toothbrush and gargled with medicated mouthrinses.
Height	5 feet, 10 inches	
Weight	180 pounds	
BP	115/95 mm Hg	
Chief Complaint	*"Why are my bottom eyeteeth sensitive at the gumline when I drink fresh coffee?"*	
Medical History	Smokes and has high blood pressure controlled with medication	
Current Medications	Diuretics	
Social History	Writer of science fiction	

1. What is the CORRECT angle classification of malocclusion on the patient's posterior dentition on the right side?
   A. Class I
   B. Class II, Division I
   C. Class II, Division II
   D. Class III

2. What other occlusal evaluation notes can be made regarding the right side of the dentition?
   A. Severe crossbite
   B. Open bite
   C. Severe overjet
   D. End-to-end bite

3. What may be occurring on the patient's mandibular teeth to make them sensitive to hot fluids?
   A. Erosion
   B. Abfraction
   C. Pulpitis
   D. Toothbrush abrasion

4. What is the correct term used for grinding the teeth?
   A. Clenching
   B. Xerostomia
   C. Bruxism
   D. Passive eruption

5. What part of the anatomy of each sensitive tooth is FIRST lost with grinding?
   A. Fossae
   B. Pits
   C. Grooves
   D. Cusps

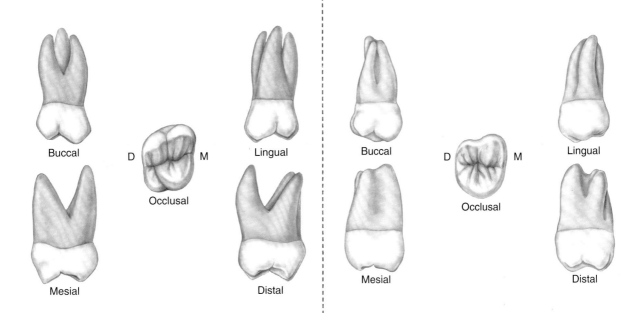

Buccal

D ⏐ M
Occlusal

Lingual

Mesial

Distal

Buccal

D ⏐ M
Occlusal

Lingual

Mesial

Distal

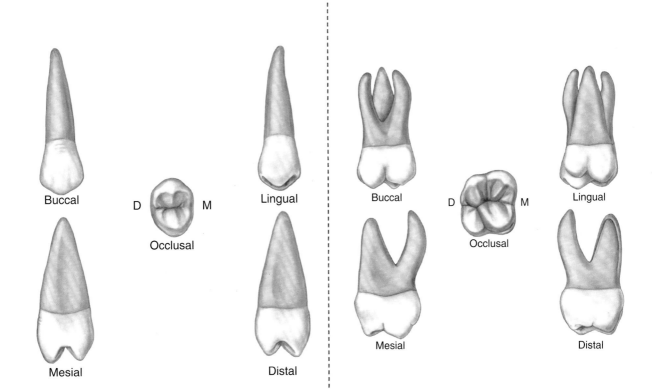

Buccal

D ⏐ M
Occlusal

Lingual

Mesial

Distal

Buccal

D ⏐ M
Occlusal

Lingual

Mesial

Distal

Maxillary Right Third Molar (Heart-shaped Occlusal Outline)

CHARACTERISTICS:

Universal Number: #1 **International Number:** #18
Eruption: 17-21
Root completion: 18-25
General crown features: Occlusal table with marginal ridges and cusps with tips, inclined planes, ridges, grooves, fossae, and pits
Specific crown features: Smaller crown than second and variable in form. Heart-shaped or rhomboidal crown outline, with three or four cusps. Buccal cervical ridge
Height of Contour: Buccal: cervical third; Lingual: middle third
Mesial contact: Middle third
Distal contact: None
Distinguishing right from left: Distobuccal cusp shorter than mesiobuccal cusp. Roots curve distally
General Root Features: Three roots
Specific Root features: Less divergent roots. Usually fused roots, curving distally

Maxillary Right Second Molar (Rhomboidal Crown Outline)

CHARACTERISTICS:

Universal Number: #2 **International Number:** #17
Eruption: 12-13
Root completion: 14-16
General crown features: Occlusal table with marginal ridges and cusps with tips, inclined planes, ridges, grooves, fossae, and pits
Specific crown features: Smaller crown than first. Heart-shaped or rhomboidal crown outline, with three or four cusps. Less prominent oblique ridge. Mesiobuccal cusp longer than distobuccal cusp. Distolingual cusp smaller than on first or absent. No fifth cusp. Buccal cervical ridge
Height of Contour: Buccal: cervical third; Lingual: middle third
Mesial contact: Middle third
Distal contact: Middle third
Distinguishing right from left: Mesiolingual cusp outline longer and larger but not as sharp as distolingual cusp outline
General Root features: Three roots
Specific Root Features: Furcations. Root trunks and root concavities. Less divergent roots

Maxillary Right First Molar

CHARACTERISTICS:

Universal Number: #3 **International Number:** #16
Eruption: 6-7
Root completion: 9-10
General crown features: Occlusal table with marginal ridges and cusps with tips, inclined planes, ridges, grooves, fossae, and pits
Specific crown features: Largest tooth in arch and largest crown in dentition. Prominent oblique ridge. Four major cusps, with buccal cusps almost equal in height. Fifth minor cusp of Carabelli associated with mesiolingual cusp. Buccal cervical ridge
Height of Contour: Buccal: cervical third; Lingual: middle third
Mesial contact: Junction of occlusal and middle thirds
Distal contact: Middle third
Distinguishing right from left: Mesiolingual cusp outline longer and larger but not as sharp as distolingual cusp outline
General Root features: Three roots
Specific Root Features: Furcations well removed from CEJ. Root trunks and root concavities. Divergent roots

Maxillary Right Second Premolar

CHARACTERISTICS:

Universal Number: #4 **International Number:** #15
Eruption: 10-12
Root completion: 12-14
General crown features: Occlusal table with marginal ridges and cusps with tips, ridges, inclined planes, grooves, fossae, pits
Specific crown features: Smaller than first. Two cusps same length. Short central groove, with increased supplemental grooves. No mesial surface features like first. Buccal ridge
Height of Contour: Buccal: cervical third; Lingual: middle third
Mesial contact: Just cervical to the junction of occlusal and middle thirds
Distal contact: Just cervical to the junction of occlusal and middle thirds
Distinguishing right from left: Lingual cusp to offset to the mesial
General root features: Single root
Specific root features: . Elliptic on cross section. Proximal root concavities

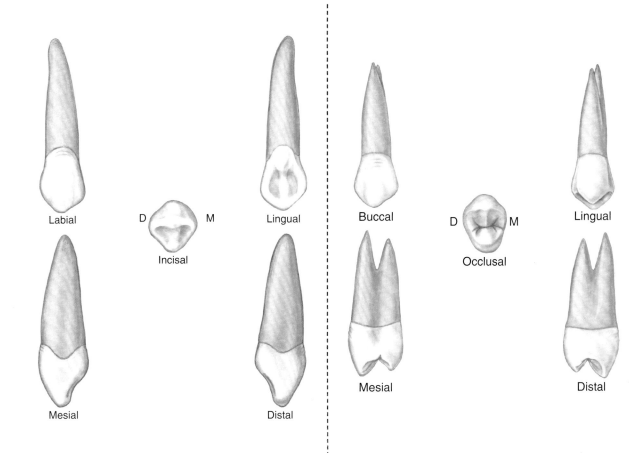

Labial   D   M   Lingual

Incisal

Mesial   Distal

Buccal   D   M   Lingual

Occlusal

Mesial   Distal

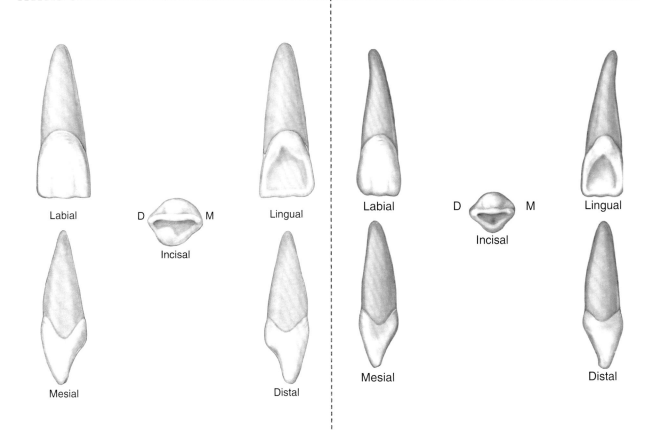

Labial   D   M   Lingual

Incisal

Mesial   Distal

Labial   D   M   Lingual

Incisal

Mesial   Distal

Maxillary Right First Premolar

CHARACTERISTICS:

Universal Number: #5 **International Number:** #14
Eruption 10-11
Root completion: 12-13
General crown features: Occlusal table with marginal ridges and cusps with tips, ridges, inclined planes, grooves, fossae, pits
Specific crown features: Larger than second. Buccal cusp longer of two cusps. Long central groove. Mesial surface features unlike second. Buccal ridge
Height of Contour: Buccal: cervical third; Lingual: middle third
Mesial contact: Just cervical to the junction of occlusal and middle thirds
Distal contact: Just cervical to the junction of occlusal and middle thirds
Distinguishing right from left: Longer mesial cusp slope than distal cusp slope, with mesial features: deeper CEJ curvature, marginal groove, developmental depression
General root features: Two roots with root trunk
Specific root features: Elliptic on cross section. Proximal root concavities

Maxillary Right Canine

CHARACTERISTICS:

Universal Number: #6 **International Number:** #13
Eruption: 11-12
Root completion: 13-15
General crown features: Single cusp with tip and slopes, labial ridge, cingulum, lingual ridge, marginal ridges, and lingual fossae
Specific crown features: Longest tooth in arch. Prominent lingual surface. Sharp cusp tip
Height of contour: Labial: cervical third; Lingual: middle third
Mesial contact: Junction of incisal third and middle thirds
Distal contact: Middle third
Distinguishing right from left: Shorter mesial cusp slope than distal cusp slope, with more pronounced mesial CEJ curvature. More cervical contact on distal. Shorter distal outline than mesial outline on labial view and with depression between the distal contact and CEJ
General root features: Long, thick single root
Specific root features: Oval on cross section. Proximal root concavities. Blunt root apex

Maxillary Right Lateral Incisor

CHARACTERISTICS:

Universal Number: #7 **International Number:** #12
Eruption: 8-9
Root completion: 11
General crown features: Incisal ridge, incisal angles, cingulum, marginal ridges, lingual fossa
Specific crown features: Greatest crown variation. Like a smaller central. Pronounced lingual surface, with centered cingulum and prominent marginal ridges
Height of contour: Cervical third
Mesial contact: Incisal third
Distal contact: Middle third
Distinguishing right from left: Sharper mesioincisal angle and rounder distoincisal angle. More pronounced mesial CEJ curvature
General root features: Single root
Specific root features: Oval in cross section. Same or longer than central but thinner. Overall conical shape. No proximal root concavities. Root curves distally, with sharp apex

Maxillary Right Central Incisor

CHARACTERISTICS:

Universal Number: #8 **International Number:** #11
Eruption: 7-8
Root completion: 10
General crown features: Incisal ridge, incisal angles, cingulum, marginal ridges, lingual fossa
Specific crown features: Widest crown mesiodistally. Greatest CEJ curve and height of contour. Pronounced distal offset cingulum and marginal ridges, with wide and deep lingual fossa
Height of contour: Cervical third
Mesial contact: Incisal third
Distal contact: Junction of incisal and middle thirds
Distinguishing right from left: Sharper mesioincisal angle and rounder distoincisal angle. More pronounced mesial CEJ curvature
General root features: Single root
Specific root features: Triangular in cross section. Overall conical shape. No proximal root concavities. Rounded apex

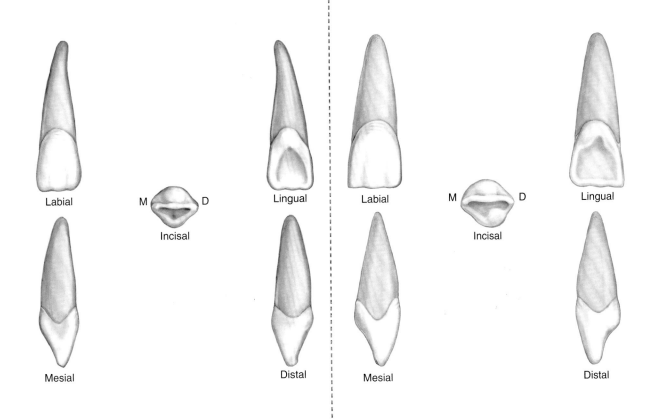

Labial   M ⌣ D   Lingual

Incisal

Mesial   Distal

Labial   M ⌣ D   Lingual

Incisal

Mesial   Distal

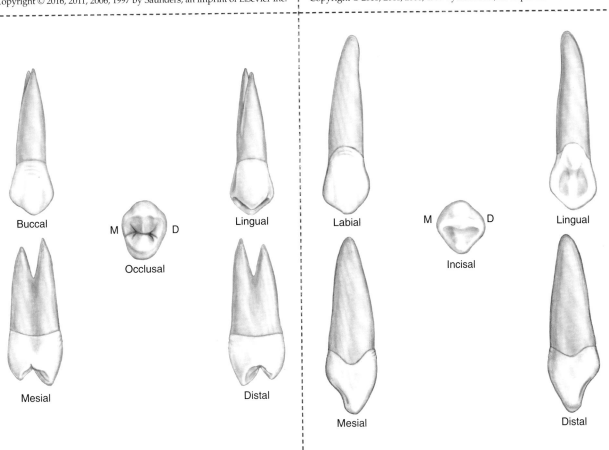

Buccal   M ⌣ D   Lingual

Occlusal

Mesial   Distal

Labial   M ⌣ D   Lingual

Incisal

Mesial   Distal

Maxillary Left Central Incisor

CHARACTERISTICS:

Universal Number: #9 International Number: #21
Eruption: 7-8
Root completion: 10
General crown features: Incisal ridge, incisal angles, cingulum, marginal ridges, lingual fossa
Specific crown features: Widest crown mesiodistally. Greatest CEJ curve and height of contour. Pronounced distal offset cingulum and marginal ridges, with wide and deep lingual fossa
Height of contour: Cervical third
Mesial contact: Incisal third
Distal contact: Junction of incisal and middle thirds
Distinguishing right from left: Sharper mesioincisal angle and rounder distoincisal angle. More pronounced mesial CEJ curvature
General root features: Single root
Specific root features: Triangular in cross section. Overall conical shape. No proximal root concavities. Rounded apex

Maxillary Left Lateral Incisor

CHARACTERISTICS:

Universal Number: #10 International Number: #22
Eruption: 8-9
Root completion: 11
General crown features: Incisal ridge, incisal angles, cingulum, marginal ridges, lingual fossa
Specific crown features: Greatest crown variation. Like a smaller central. Pronounced lingual surface, with centered cingulum and prominent marginal ridges
Height of contour: Cervical third
Mesial contact: Incisal third
Distal contact: Middle third
Distinguishing right from left: Sharper mesioincisal angle and rounder distoincisal angle. More pronounced mesial CEJ curvature
General root features: Single root
Specific root features: Oval in cross section. Same or longer than central but thinner. Overall conical shape. No proximal root concavities. Root curves distally, with sharp apex

Maxillary Left Canine

CHARACTERISTICS:

Universal Number: #11 International Number: #23
Eruption: 11-12
Root completion: 13-15
General crown features: Single cusp with tip and slopes, labial ridge, cingulum, lingual ridge, marginal ridges, and lingual fossae
Specific crown features: Longest tooth in arch. Prominent lingual surface. Sharp cusp tip
Height of contour: Labial: cervical third; Lingual: middle third
Mesial contact: Junction of incisal third and middle thirds
Distal contact: Middle third
Distinguishing right from left: Shorter mesial cusp slope than distal cusp slope, with more pronounced mesial CEJ curvature. More cervical contact on distal. Shorter distal outline than mesial outline on labial view and with depression between the distal contact and CEJ
General root features: Long, thick single root
Specific root features: Oval on cross section. Proximal root concavities. Blunt root apex

Maxillary Left First Premolar

CHARACTERISTICS:

Universal Number: #12 International Number: #24
Eruption: 10-11
Root completion: 12-13
General crown features: Occlusal table with marginal ridges and cusps and with tips, ridges, inclined planes, grooves, fossae, pits
Specific crown features: Larger than second. Buccal cusp longer of two cusps. Long central groove. Mesial surface features unlike second. Buccal ridge
Height of Contour: Buccal: cervical third; Lingual: middle third
Mesial contact: Just cervical to the junction of occlusal and middle thirds
Distal contact: Just cervical to the junction of occlusal and middle thirds
Distinguishing right from left: Longer mesial cusp slope than distal cusp slope, with mesial features: deeper CEJ curvature, marginal groove, developmental depression
General root features: Two roots with root trunk
Specific root features: Elliptic on cross section. Proximal root concavities

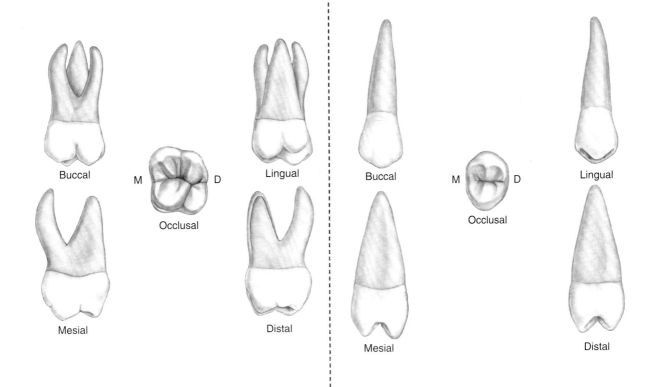

Buccal

M   Occlusal   D

Lingual

Mesial

Distal

Buccal

M   Occlusal   D

Lingual

Mesial

Distal

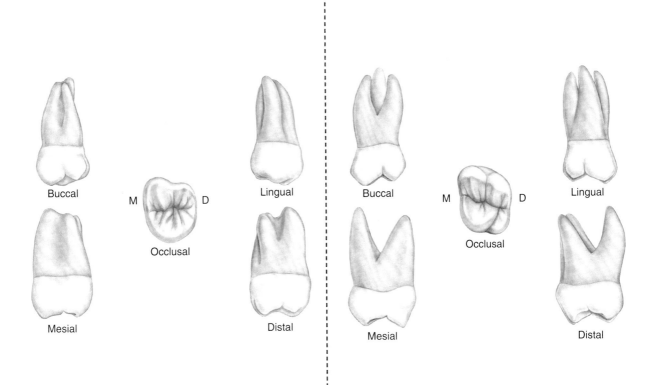

Buccal

M   Occlusal   D

Lingual

Mesial

Distal

Buccal

M   Occlusal   D

Lingual

Mesial

Distal

Maxillary Left Second Premolar

CHARACTERISTICS:

Universal Number: #13 **International Number:** #25
Eruption: 10-12
Root completion: 12-14
General crown features: Occlusal table with marginal ridges and cusps with tips, ridges, inclined planes, grooves, fossae, pits
Specific crown features: Smaller than first. Two cusps same length. Short central groove, with increased supplemental grooves. No mesial surface features like first. Buccal ridge
Height of Contour: Buccal: cervical third; Lingual: middle third
Mesial contact: Just cervical to the junction of occlusal and middle thirds
Distal contact: Just cervical to the junction of occlusal and middle thirds
Distinguishing right from left: Lingual cusp to offset to the mesial
General root features: Single root
Specific root features: Elliptic on cross section. Proximal root concavities

Maxillary Left First Molar

CHARACTERISTICS:

Universal Number: #14 **International Number:** #26
Eruption: 6-7
Root completion: 9-10
General crown features: Occlusal table with marginal ridges and cusps with tips, inclined planes, ridges, grooves, fossae, and pits. Buccal cervical ridge
Specific crown features: Largest tooth in arch, largest crown in dentition. Four major cusps, with buccal cusps almost equal in height. Fifth minor cusp of Carabelli associated with mesiolingual cusp and prominent oblique ridge
Height of Contour: Buccal: cervical third; Lingual: middle third
Mesial contact: Junction of occlusal and middle thirds
Distal contact: Middle third
Distinguishing right from left: Mesiolingual cusp outline longer and larger but not as sharp as distolingual cusp outline
General Root features: Three roots
Specific Root Features: Furcations well removed from CEJ. Root trunks and root concavities. Divergent roots

Maxillary Left Second Molar (Rhomboidal Crown Outline)

CHARACTERISTICS:

Universal Number: #15 **International Number:** #27
Eruption: 12-13
Root completion: 14-16
General crown features: Occlusal table with marginal ridges and cusps with tips, inclined planes, ridges, grooves, fossae, and pits
Specific crown features: Smaller crown than first. Heart-shaped or rhomboidal crown outline, with three or four cusps. Less prominent oblique ridge. Mesiobuccal cusp longer than distobuccal cusp. Distolingual cusp smaller than on first or absent. No fifth cusp. Buccal cervical ridge
Height of Contour: Buccal: cervical third; Lingual: middle third
Mesial contact: Middle third
Distal contact: Middle third
Distinguishing right from left: Mesiolingual cusp outline longer and larger but not as sharp as distolingual cusp outline
General Root features: Three roots
Specific Root Features: Furcations. Root trunks and root concavities. Less divergent roots

Maxillary Left Third Molar (Heart-shaped Occlusal Outline)

CHARACTERISTICS:

Universal Number: #16 **International Number:** #28
Eruption: 17-21
Root completion: 18-25
General crown features: Occlusal table with marginal ridges and cusps with tips, inclined planes, ridges, grooves, fossae, and pits
Specific crown features: Smaller crown than second and variable in form. Heart-shaped or rhomboidal crown outline, with three or four cusps. Buccal cervical ridge
Height of Contour: Buccal: cervical third; Lingual: middle third
Mesial contact: Middle third
Distal contact: None
Distinguishing right from left: Distobuccal cusp shorter than mesiobuccal cusp. Roots curve distally
General Root Features: Three roots
Specific Root features: Less divergent roots. Usually fused roots, curving distally

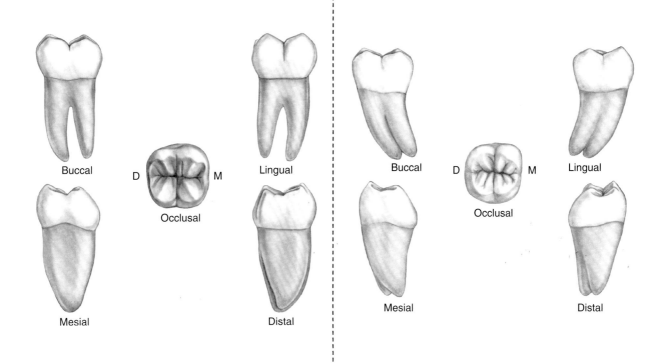

Buccal

D Occlusal M

Lingual

Mesial

Distal

Buccal

D Occlusal M

Lingual

Mesial

Distal

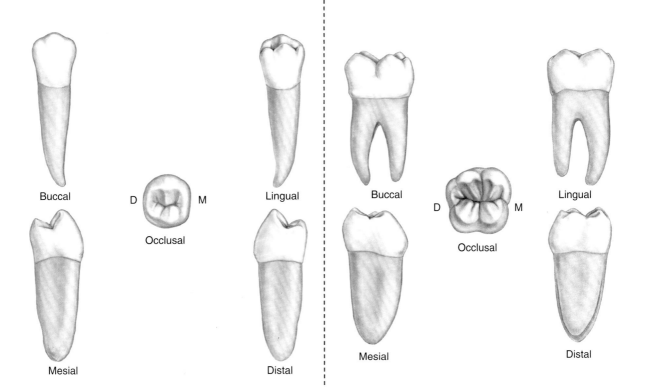

Buccal

D Occlusal M

Lingual

Mesial

Distal

Buccal

D Occlusal M

Lingual

Mesial

Distal

Mandibular Left Third Molar

CHARACTERISTICS:

Universal Number: #17 International Number: #38
Eruption: 17-21
Root completion: 18-25
General crown features: Occlusal table with marginal ridges and cusps with tips, inclined planes, ridges, grooves, fossae, and pits
Specific crown features: Smaller crown than second
Height of Contour: Buccal: cervical third; Lingual: middle third
Mesial contact: Cervical third
Distal contact: None
Distinguishing right from left: Wider buccolingually on mesial than on distal
General root features: Two roots
Specific root features: Fused roots, irregularly curved, with sharp apices

Mandibular Left Second Molar

CHARACTERISTICS:

Universal Number: #18 International Number: #37
Eruption: 11-13
Root completion: 14-15
General crown features: Occlusal table with marginal ridges and cusps with tips, inclined planes, ridges, grooves, fossae, and pits
Specific crown features: Smaller crown than first. Four cusps with cross-shaped groove pattern
Height of Contour: Buccal: cervical third; Lingual: middle third
Mesial contact: Middle third
Distal contact: Middle third
Distinguishing right from left: Difference in height of contour for buccal and lingual from each proximal surface and wider on the mesial than distal
General root features: Two roots
Specific root features: Furcations closer to CEJ. Root trunks and root concavities. Less divergent roots

Mandibular Left First Molar

CHARACTERISTICS:

Universal Number: #19 International Number: #36
Eruption: 6-7
Root completion: 9-10
General crown features: Occlusal table with marginal ridges and cusps with tips, inclined planes, ridges, grooves, fossae, and pits
Specific crown features: First permanent tooth to erupt. Widest crown mesiodistally of dentition. Five cusps with Y-shaped groove pattern. Buccal groove possibly ending in buccal pit
Height of Contour: Buccal: cervical third; Lingual: middle third
Mesial contact: Junction of occlusal and middle thirds
Distal contact: Junction of occlusal and middle thirds
Distinguishing right from left: Distal cusp is smallest with sharp cusp
General root features: Two roots
Specific root features: Furcations well removed from the CEJ. Root trunks and root concavities. Divergent roots

Mandibular Left Second Premolar
(Three-Cusp Type)

CHARACTERISTICS:

Universal Number: #20 International Number: #35
Eruption: 11-12
Root completion: 13-14
General crown features: Occlusal table with marginal ridges and cusps with tips, ridges, inclined planes, grooves, fossae, pits. Buccal ridge
Specific crown features: Larger than first. Usually three cusps with Y-shaped groove pattern or two cusps with H or U-shaped groove pattern. Increased supplemental grooves
Height of Contour: Buccal: cervical third; Lingual: middle third
Mesial contact: Just cervical to the junction of occlusal and middle thirds
Distal contact: Just cervical to the junction of occlusal and middle thirds
Distinguishing right from left: Distal marginal ridge more cervically located, with more occlusal surface visible from distal view
General root features: Single root
Specific root features: Oval or elliptic on cross section. Proximal root concavities

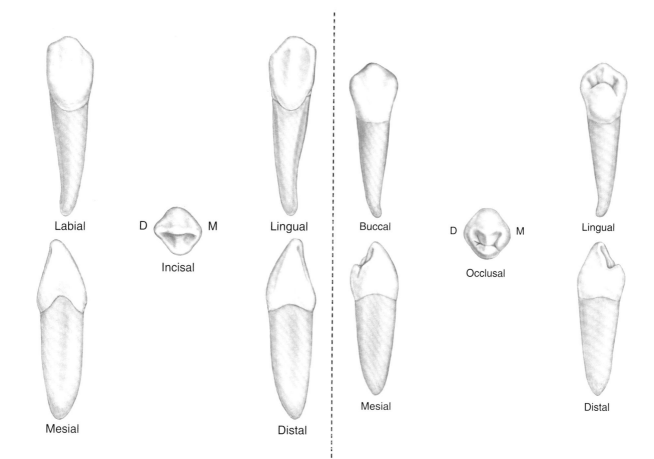

Labial   D   M   Lingual

Incisal

Mesial   Distal

Buccal   D   M   Lingual

Occlusal

Mesial   Distal

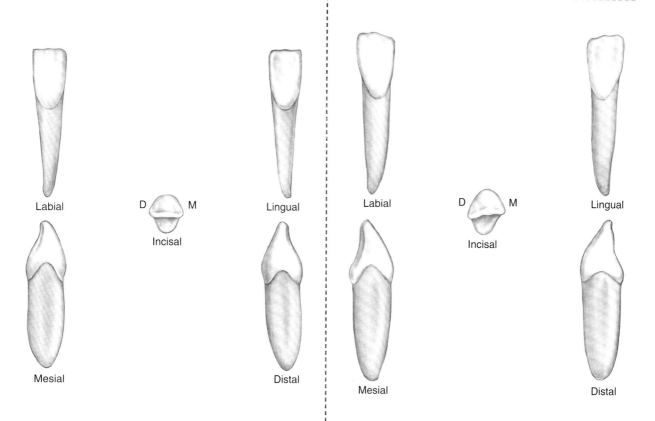

Labial   D   M   Lingual

Incisal

Mesial   Distal

Labial   D   M   Lingual

Incisal

Mesial   Distal

Mandibular Left First Premolar

CHARACTERISTICS:

Universal Number: #21 **International Number:** #34
Eruption: 10-12
Root completion: 12-13
General crown features: Occlusal table with marginal ridges and cusps with tips, ridges, inclined planes, grooves, fossae, pits
Specific crown features: Smaller than second. Smaller lingual cusp of two cusps. Mesial surface features. Buccal ridge
Height of Contour: Buccal: cervical third; Lingual: middle third
Mesial contact: Just cervical to the junction of occlusal and middle thirds
Distal contact: Just cervical to the junction of occlusal and middle thirds
Distinguishing right from left: Shorter mesial cusp slope than distal cusp slope, with mesial surface features: deeper mesial CEJ curvature and mesiolingual groove
General root features: Single root
Specific root features: Oval or elliptic on cross section. Proximal root concavities

Mandibular Left Canine

CHARACTERISTICS:

Universal Number: #22 **International Number:** #33
Eruption: 9-10
Root completion: 12-14
General crown features: Single cusp with tip and slopes, labial ridge, cingulum, lingual ridge, marginal ridges, and lingual fossae
Specific crown features: Longest tooth in arch. Less pronounced lingual surface. Less sharp cusp tip
Height of contour: Labial: cervical third; Lingual: middle third
Mesial contact: Incisal third
Distal contact: Junction of incisal and middle thirds
Distinguishing right from left: Shorter mesial cusp slope than distal cusp slope, with more pronounced mesial CEJ curvature. More cervical contact on distal. Shorter and rounder distal outline than mesial outline on labial view, with a shorter mesial slope than distal cusp slope
General root features: Long, thick single root
Specific root features: Oval on cross section. Proximal root concavities, with developmental depressions on mesial and distal, giving tooth double-rooted appearance. Pointed apex

Mandibular Left Lateral Incisor

CHARACTERISTICS:

Universal Number: #23 **International Number:** #32
Eruption: 7-8
Root completion: 10
General crown features: Incisal ridge, incisal angles, cingulum, marginal ridges, lingual fossa
Specific crown features: Like a larger mandibular central. Not symmetric. Appears twisted distally. Small, distally placed cingulum, with mesial marginal ridge longer than distal marginal ridge
Height of contour: Cervical third
Mesial contact: Incisal third
Distal contact: Incisal third
Distinguishing right from left: Sharper mesioincisal angle and rounder distoincisal angle. More pronounced mesial CEJ curvature
General root features: Single root
Specific root features: Elliptic on cross section. Root is longer than the crown. Pronounced proximal root concavities can give double-rooted appearance

Mandibular Left Central Incisor

CHARACTERISTICS:

Universal Number: #24 **International Number:** #31
Eruption: 6-7
Root completion: 9
General crown features: Incisal ridge, incisal angles, cingulum, marginal ridges, lingual fossa
Specific crown features: Smallest and simplest tooth. Symmetric. Small centered cingulum, with less pronounced marginal ridges and lingual fossa
Height of contour: Cervical third
Mesial contact: Incisal third
Distal contact: Incisal third
Distinguishing right from left: Sharper mesioincisal angle and rounder distoincisal angle. More pronounced mesial CEJ curvature
General root features: Single root
Specific root features: Elliptic on cross section. Root is longer than the crown. Pronounced proximal root concavities can give double-rooted appearance

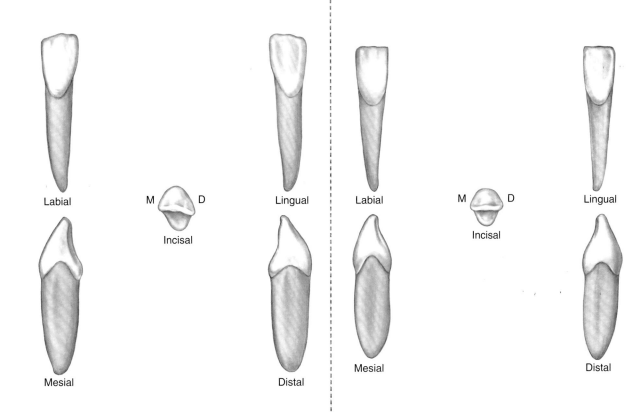

Labial

M ◠ D
Incisal

Lingual

Mesial

Distal

Labial

M ◠ D
Incisal

Lingual

Mesial

Distal

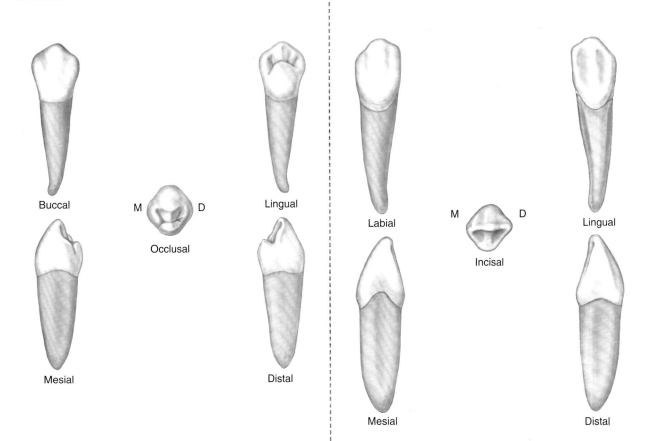

Buccal

M ◠ D
Occlusal

Lingual

Mesial

Distal

Labial

M ◠ D
Incisal

Lingual

Mesial

Distal

Mandibular Right Central Incisor

CHARACTERISTICS:

Universal Number: #25 **International Number:** #41
Eruption: 6-7
Root completion: 9
General crown features: Incisal ridge, incisal angles, cingulum, marginal ridges, lingual fossa
Specific crown features: Smallest and simplest tooth. Symmetric. Small centered cingulum, with less pronounced marginal ridges and lingual fossa
Height of contour: Cervical third
Mesial contact: Incisal third
Distal contact: Incisal third
Distinguishing right from left: Sharper mesioincisal angle and rounder distoincisal angle. More pronounced mesial CEJ curvature
General root features: Single root
Specific root features: Elliptic on cross section. Root is longer than the crown. Pronounced proximal root concavities can give double-rooted appearance

Mandibular Right Lateral Incisor

CHARACTERISTICS:

Universal Number: #26 **International Number:** #42
Eruption: 7-8
Root completion: 10
General crown features: Incisal ridge, incisal angles, cingulum, marginal ridges, lingual fossa
Specific crown features: Like a larger mandibular central, Not symmetric. Appears twisted distally. Small, distally placed cingulum, with mesial marginal ridge longer than distal marginal ridge
Height of contour: Cervical third
Mesial contact: Incisal third
Distal contact: Incisal third
Distinguishing right from left: Sharper mesioincisal angle and rounder distoincisal angle. More pronounced mesial CEJ curvature
General root features: Single root
Specific root features: Elliptic on cross section. Root is longer than the crown. Proximal root concavities can give double-rooted appearance

Mandibular Right Canine

CHARACTERISTICS:

Universal Number: #27 **International Number:** #43
Eruption: 9-10
Root completion: 12-14
General crown features: Single cusp with tip and slopes, labial ridge, cingulum, lingual ridge, marginal ridges, and lingual fossae
Specific crown features: Longest tooth in arch. Less pronounced lingual surface. Less sharp cusp tip
Height of contour: Labial: cervical third; Lingual: middle third
Mesial contact: Incisal third
Distal contact: Junction of incisal and middle thirds
Distinguishing right from left: Shorter mesial cusp slope than distal cusp slope, with more pronounced mesial CEJ curvature. More cervical contact on distal. Shorter and rounder distal outline than mesial outline on labial view, with a shorter mesial slope than distal slope
General root features: Long, thick single root
Specific root features: Oval on cross section. Proximal root concavities, with developmental depressions on mesial and distal giving tooth double-rooted appearance. Pointed apex

Mandibular Right First Premolar

CHARACTERISTICS:

Universal Number: #28 **International Number:** #44
Eruption: 10-12
Root completion: 12-13
General crown features: Occlusal table with marginal ridges and cusps with tips, ridges, inclined planes, grooves, fossae, pits.
Specific crown features: Smaller than second. Smaller lingual cusp of two cusps. Mesial surface features. Buccal ridge
Height of Contour: Buccal: cervical third; Lingual: middle third
Mesial contact: Just cervical to the junction of occlusal and middle thirds
Distal contact: Just cervical to the junction of occlusal and middle thirds
Distinguishing right from left: Shorter mesial cusp slope than distal cusp slope, with mesial surface features: deeper mesial CEJ curvature and mesiolingual groove
General root features: Single root
Specific root features: Oval or elliptic on cross section. Proximal root concavities

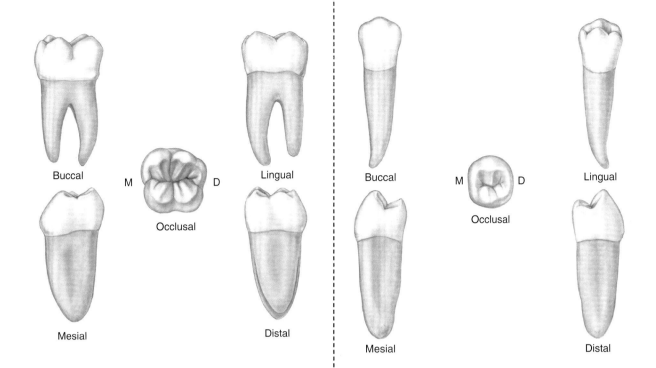

Buccal

M Occlusal D

Lingual

Mesial

Distal

Buccal

M Occlusal D

Lingual

Mesial

Distal

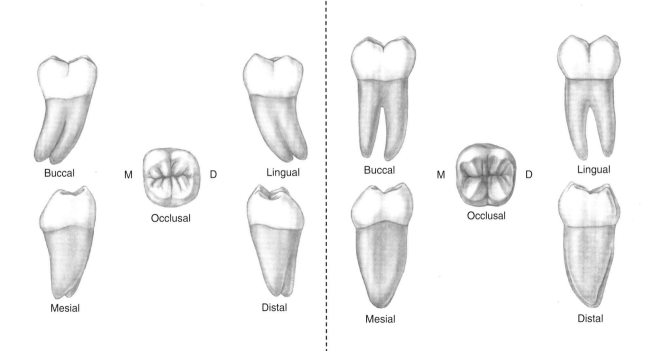

Buccal

M Occlusal D

Lingual

Mesial

Distal

Buccal

M Occlusal D

Lingual

Mesial

Distal

Mandibular Right Second Premolar (Three-Cusp Type)

CHARACTERISTICS:

Universal Number: #29 **International Number:** #45
Eruption: 11-12
Root completion: 13-14
General crown features: Occlusal table with marginal ridges and cusps with tips, ridges, inclined planes, grooves, fossae, pits
Specific crown features: Larger than first. Usually three cusps with Y-shaped groove pattern or two cusps with H or U-shaped groove pattern. Increased supplemental grooves. Buccal ridge
Height of Contour: Buccal: cervical third; Lingual: middle third
Mesial contact: Just cervical to the junction of occlusal and middle thirds
Distal contact: Just cervical to the junction of occlusal and middle thirds
Distinguishing right from left: Distal marginal ridge more cervically located, thus more occlusal surface visible from distal view
General root features: Single root
Specific root features: Oval or elliptic on cross section. Proximal root concavities

Mandibular Right First Molar

CHARACTERISTICS:

Universal Number: #30 **International Number:** #46
Eruption: 6-7
Root completion: 9-10
General crown features: Occlusal table with marginal ridges and cusps with tips, inclined planes, ridges, grooves, fossae, and pits
Specific crown features: First permanent tooth to erupt. Widest crown mesiodistally of dentition. Five cusps with Y-shaped groove pattern. Buccal groove possibly ending in buccal pit
Height of Contour: Buccal: cervical third; Lingual: middle third
Mesial contact: Junction of occlusal and middle thirds
Distal contact: Junction of occlusal and middle thirds
Distinguishing right from left: Distal cusp is smallest and has a sharp cusp
General root features: Two roots
Specific root features: Furcations well removed from the CEJ. Root trunks and root concavities. Divergent roots

Mandibular Right Second Molar

CHARACTERISTICS:

Universal Number: #31 **International Number:** #47
Eruption: 11-13
Root completion: 14-15
General crown features: Occlusal table with marginal ridges and cusps with tips, inclined planes, ridges, grooves, fossae, and pits
Specific crown features: Smaller crown than first. Four cusps with cross-shaped groove pattern
Height of Contour: Buccal: cervical third; Lingual: middle third
Mesial contact: Middle third
Distal contact: Middle third
Distinguishing right from left: Difference in height of contour for buccal and lingual from each proximal surface and wider on the mesial than distal
General root features: Two roots
Specific root features: Furcations closer to CEJ. Root trunks and root concavities. Less divergent roots

Mandibular Right Third Molar

CHARACTERISTICS:

Universal Number: #32 **International Number:** #48
Eruption: 17-21
Root completion: 18-25
General crown features: Occlusal table with marginal ridges and cusps with tips, inclined planes, ridges, grooves, fossae, and pits
Specific crown features: Smaller crown than second
Height of Contour: Buccal: cervical third; Lingual: middle third
Mesial contact: Cervical third
Distal contact: None
Distinguishing right from left: Wider buccolingually on mesial than on distal
General root features: Two roots
Specific root features: Fused roots, irregularly curved, with sharp apices